Healthy MADE SIMPLE

BIRGITTE HAANING CHRISTENSEN

Healthy Made Simple

Published by Birgitte Haaning Christensen
bc@mygoodwitch.com
www.mygoodwitch.com

Produced by Create and Blossom
712 Austin Avenue
Waco, TX 76701
www.createandblossomstudios.com

ISBN: 978-1-945304-72-9 hardcover
ISBN: 978-1-945304-36-1 Paperback
ISBN: 978-1-945304-76-7 eBook
Library of Congress Control Number: 2024908155

First Edition

“

There is so much more to a healthy lifestyle than food and exercise, and it is really not very complicated.

~Birgitte Haaning Christensen

TABLE OF CONTENTS

Dedication **1**

Introduction **3**

My Journey to Better Health **5**

The Story of My Ancestors **9**

Section One GOOD TO KNOW

Chapter One **15**

HEALTHY MADE SIMPLE 17

Chapter Two **19**

THE HUMAN CELL 21

Cells Becomes Systems 22

Chapter Three **25**

ENERGIES AND RHYTHMS 27

The Main Rhythm 27

The Circadian Rhythm 29

The Law of the 5 Elements 31

Chapter Four **35**

OXIDATIVE STRESS 37

What Is Oxidative Stress? 37

How Does Oxidative Stress Harm Us 38

What Can You Do 39

Chapter Five **41**

INFLAMMATION 43

What Causes Inflammation 43

How To Fight Inflammation 44

Chapter Six **47**

GUT HEALTH 49

Drink Enough Water 50

Physical Activity 51

Chapter Seven **53**
PH BALANCE 55
Chapter Eight **59**
MY SEVEN STEPS 61
Food 62
Water 63
Sleep 64
Exercise 65
Fresh Air 66
Grounding 66
Silence 67
Gratitude 68

Section Two MINDFUL EATING

Chapter Nine **73**
A BALANCED DIET 75
Our Food 75
You Can Eat Almost Anything 76
The Mindful Eating Circle 77
Vegetables - 2 ½ - 3 cups 78
Fruit & Berry - 1 cup 78
Protein - 7 - 12 oz 78
Healthy Fats - 1 - 1 ¼ cup 79
Carbs (starches) - ½ - ¾ cup 79
The Key Is Fiber 80
Benefits Of Fiber 80
Carbohydrates 82
Processed Food 83
Reboot Your Sugar Intake 85
Why Is Sugar So Addictive 86
The Different Types Of Sugar 87
What Does Sugar Actually Do To Your Body 89

Dairy 91
Gluten 94
Fat & Fatty Acids 96
Processed Fatty Acids 97
The Healthy Fatty Acids..98

Section Three MINDFUL LIVING

Chapter Ten 107
OUTDOORS 109
Fresh Air 109
Grounding 111
How To Do It 112
Benefits Of Grounding 113
Tools used for grounding..114
Exercise 115

Chapter Eleven 119
SELF AWARENESS 121
The 4 Levels Of Awareness...123
Coherence 124
Gratitude 125
The Line Of Decision 125
Your Inner Child..128
I am's 128
Living The 4 Levels Of Awareness...129
Level 1 - Low Awareness 131
Level 2 - Some Awareness 135
Level 3 - High Awareness 139
Level 4 - Highest Awareness 143

Chapter Twelve 147
DETOX 149
My Simple Detox Tools 150
Oil Pulling 151

Step By Step 153
Detox Drinks 154
How To Do It 157
Dry Brushing 158
How To Dry Brush 161
Why Dry Brush 161
Foot Baths 163
Supplements, Herbs And Plants 167
Healthy Living 171
Chapter Thirteen 173
STRESS MANAGEMENT 175
Time Management 180
Benefits Of Good Time Management 181
Stress And Time Management Tools 182
Declutter And Organize 188
Silence 190
Gratitude 191
How Do You Do It 193
Closing 195
Disclaimer 199
Links page 200

Dedication

I dedicate this book to the love of my life, my dear husband, and business partner, Andy. Thank you for always believing in me and encouraging me to get this book finished. I don't know what I would do without you. And to my two beautiful and wonderful kids for your patience - willing or unwilling - with all the different approaches to healthy living I put you through while you were growing up. And now as grown ups your support and encouragement mean the world to me.

Thank you to my dear friends Susanne and Kirsten who taught me so much over the years. You have both always been there for me with answers and guidance. I am forever grateful for your friendship. And to my mentor, Frede Damgaard for always being willing to teach and share your wisdom. Your support has been invaluable.

Also a huge thank you to Kennisha, Lori, Crystal and Kirsten for making this book become a reality, by helping me with accountability, editing and design. You have no idea how much you mean to me.

Last but not least, to my friends and family (you know who you are) who have supported me on this journey, you have a special place in my heart. Thank you

This book is for you who want a better quality of life; to live stressless and in total balance with yourself and your loved ones. It is for you who want to be able to say no and want to be true to YOU.

Introduction

In today's world, health advice is everywhere. Diets, exercise plans, and experts all have their say, but often, they don't lead to lasting results. It's easy to get overwhelmed and confused, and a confused mind does nothing!

What if I told you there's a simpler way to be healthy? What if we looked at health as a whole – your body, mind, and spirit, and learned how they are all connected? That's what this book, "Healthy Made Simple," is all about.

I'll share my own story about why I started this journey, as well as what I've learned from years of study in holistic health. This book is intended as a reference book. It's not here to replace modern medicine but rather be a friendly guide that complements it. There is a time and place for everything. It is my passion and life's mission to help as many as possible achieve a better quality of life.

If you, like many, believe that by eating less and exercising more you will get there, now is the time to reconsider. Mental balance, positive self-awareness, gratitude, and holistic harmony are just as vital on the journey to vibrant well-being.

I love sharing what I've learned over the years because I've discovered that there are so many things, both within ourselves and in nature, that can help you achieve a better quality of life. Unfortunately, in today's fast-paced modern life, we've forgotten about these treasures.

I'm sorry to tell you this, but there's no such thing as a quick fix. Getting back to optimal health is both hard work as well as a beautiful journey. It's not about living to be 110 years old; it's about having a quality of life that lets you truly enjoy every moment.

Together, we'll embrace simplicity, letting go of confusion, blame, and guilt. We'll explore how your body can heal, your mind can find clarity, and your spirit can thrive. And of course, we'll talk about food as well. By the end, you'll be closer to optimal health, living a life that feels true to you.

Are you ready to start this journey? Let's unlock the secrets to a "Healthy Made Simple" way of living.

My Journey to Better Health

My journey to better health started because I was sick and could not get answers from modern medicine about what was wrong! I was born and raised in Denmark where I lived with my husband and two children until we had the opportunity to move to the USA in 2013.

I have been self-employed since 2000, and love being my own boss. My parents owned a jewelry store in Denmark, and as a toddler, I was often with them in the store. It is safe to say my retail gene was activated from a very young age. When they retired, I took over the store thinking this was where I was going to be for the rest of my working life. It turned out, within a few years, that this was not the case.

No diagnosis

I had been struggling with different health issues most of my life, such as dizziness, headaches, and memory problems. I was not able to figure out why! After taking different tests, the doctors never found anything wrong. Over time, I just accepted it, as many others do, thinking it was my "normal condition" and I just had to learn to live with it. Fortunately, my mother didn't agree. I was only a young teenager when she took me to a holistic practitioner in our hometown to find out what was wrong. This is when I started learning how everything in our body is connected, and how important it is to eat and live in coherence (balance) with your body.

Some of the major challenges I had at the time were Candida, digestive issues, as well as, the gallbladder and thyroid gland being out of balance. Four to six week plans were made with strict diets and a supplement regimen I had to follow. BUT, at that age you think you are immortal, and getting really sick is only for old people! Therefore, I struggled to stay on my diet 100%. There is, however, no doubt in my mind, that the seed for the Holistic approach was planted in those teenage years.

Picky eater as a child

I was always a very picky eater as a child and young adult.
For many years, the only vegetables I liked were peas and carrots! When I got home from school, I had white bread with chocolate rather than with rye bread. When starting my own family, I tried really hard to cook healthier food for them (at least I thought it was healthier). And I tried to be a better eater myself. I had to be an example for my kids, right?
However, I was still a long way from a balanced healthy and nutritious diet.

My "wake up" call

I think taking over the jewelry store from my parents added stress to the list of health issues I already was fighting. Suddenly one day I woke up on the floor of the jewelry store face down, and was rushed to the hospital. Unfortunately, they still couldn't find anything wrong, and I was sent home. After these black outs happened a couple of times, I once again decided to seek answers in the alternative world.

I found a really good Kinesiologist and was thoroughly tested. She discovered I had a lot of heavy metal in my brain and tissue, as well as intolerance for Silver, which is not the greatest when you own a jewelry store! Still I wanted to get a diagnosis from the hospital, and with my new knowledge I asked to be tested for heavy metals and silver. And finally, after so many tests in the past, they were now able to conclude the same as the Kinesiologist.

Time for a change

Now that I knew, both in my heart and my mind, what had been causing my life long health issues; my husband and I had extensive conversations about what to do next. One thing I knew for sure was I had to make a change in my work life and let go of the business my parents built that I thought was the right one for me.

Once again, the holistic approach to health and wellness caught my attention.

I knew about reflexology and Eastern medicine, and decided that would be the perfect way for me to go. I completed a two year education in reflexology, anatomy, physiology, and nutrition. What a journey.

While learning about the importance of the right foods and supplementation to your health, my personal health journey really took off. After being consistent in taking my vitamins, omegas, and probiotics for 6-9 months, I started noticing my memory improved, which helped me finish my education and the final tests. I actually now remembered what I was reading. Slowly but surely my health improved both physically and mentally. This made me realize that I had found my calling.

Slipping through the cracks

Despite my dedication to maintaining a healthy lifestyle, there have been and probably always will be moments when I find myself slipping through the cracks. It happens to the best of us. Instead of dwelling on these lapses, I've learned to acknowledge them and move forward without frustration. Life can throw unexpected curveballs, and sometimes stress or unforeseen circumstances can lead me away from my healthy habits.

There are numerous factors that can cause me to relapse into old patterns, both consciously and unconsciously. Whether it has been my busy schedule, unexpected events, moving from Denmark to the US and not knowing my new purpose, or simply a lack of motivation, I have learned to recognize when it happens. No matter how long these relapses are, they are a natural part of my journey towards optimal health. I should not be too hard on myself when they occur. What matters most is how I react when they happen. Instead of allowing myself to spiral into negativity or self-criticism, (even though it can happen for a short period of time), I choose to view them as opportunities for growth and self-improvement. By acknowledging my relapse with understanding and compassion, I can quickly realign myself with healthy habits and continue moving forward on my path to wellness.

Each relapse serves me as a reminder of the importance of consistency and mindfulness in maintaining a healthy lifestyle. By being in tune with my body, mind and spirit, I can better navigate the ups and downs of life while remaining committed to my overall well-being. So, while I still slip through the cracks from time to time, I always strive to return to my healthy habits with renewed determination and resilience.

Today, two decades later, it is my passion and life mission to help others regain balance and optimal health. And I am happy to say, I love every minute of it.

My “Healthy made Simple” lifestyle and my “Seven Steps” have helped so many to a better quality of life.

If you, like many others think - you just have to eat less and exercise more to be healthy, you are making a big mistake. Fact is, it is just as important to have a high level of self awareness, as well as mental and financial balance.

The Story of My Ancestors

Back in 2005, when I started my professional journey in the alternative world, I did not know the story of my origin. I had no idea that more than 250 years ago we had a *naturopath** in the family. A naturopath is someone that uses natural remedies to help the body heal itself. They look at the whole body, mind, and spirit, and often use several different therapies such as massage, exercises, and nutrition, and find the root cause of an illness instead of just treating the symptoms. This is exactly how I work today! Many generations back, Maren Haaning (1782-1853) practiced what we today in Denmark would refer to as a good witch.

I knew we had a book of our family tree in the Haaning family, and I was lucky enough to borrow it. I was super excited to discover Maren Haaning and her daughters were in the book.

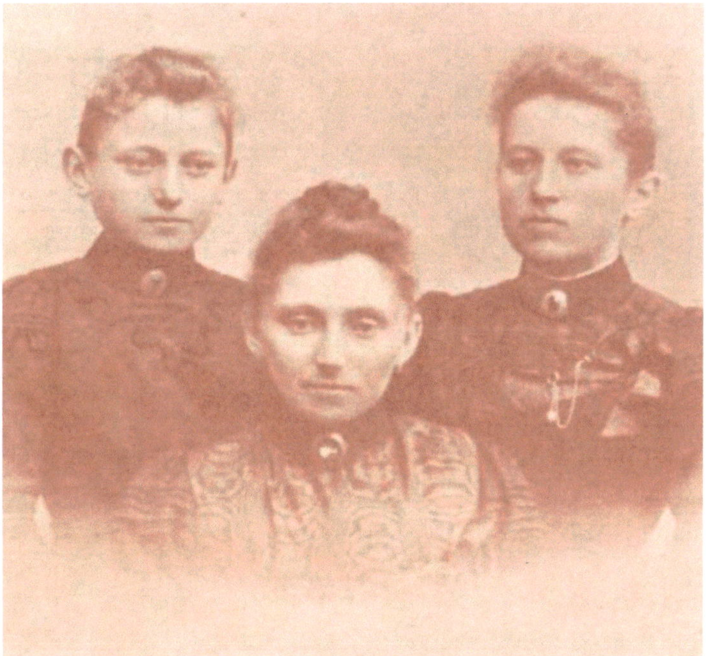

Photo of the last 3 women from the Haaning dynasty.

**A naturopath is a healthcare practitioner who emphasizes natural healing approaches, such as herbal remedies, dietary changes, and lifestyle modifications, to promote overall wellness.*

This small dynasty of naturopaths lasted 3 generations and are, in Denmark, known as the women from Vindblæs (a small town in the north eastern part of Jutland, Denmark).
Also, I found out there was a book about Maren Haaning and the 3 generations of naturopaths. How awesome is that?

I became even more excited when I discovered that the library my sister in-law was working at actually had a copy of this rare book in their storage unit. Guess what - I got for my birthday?

I felt my intuition of healing and helping others was somehow coming full circle.

Maren Haaning's story

Maren Haaning (1782-1853) was widowed at an early age and left with a poorly run farm. This forced her to find something else to do.

By coincidence she came across some old medical books, which piqued her interest, and which she later used when helping clients. Apparently, she was a natural, and had great success. In fact over time, clients sought her advice instead of going to the doctor! (she was cheaper too).

Another reason for her success was the mystique surrounding her, as she could tell where people were from and what they were suffering from, even before they had told her anything. The story goes that her son in law was making sure everything was ok in the waiting room, and carefully got the information from people, before passing it to Maren!

3 generations

Marens daughter, Maren Jensdatter (1820-1895), took over the business after her mothers passing. After all, she had all the medical books and the recipes her mother had used.

In the beginning she also relied on her mothers reputation, until she got more experience and knowledge on her own. When she died, her daughter Karen (1849-1914) and niece Maren (1872-1918) continued the business until 1918.

All three generations had problems with the authorities multiple times for giving advice without proper medical background, and because they received money for their services. However, none of them ever got convicted, because the clients never paid them directly. They put money in a jar on the kitchen counter before they left. Furthermore, they always recommended the clients to go and see the doctor too – which most of them didn't do.

To me it is mind blowing that in 2024 you still have to tell people to go and see a doctor when seeking help and advice by a "natural practitioner."

De fire kloge koner

Chresten Andersen Borup
∞
Margrethe Nielsdatter

Laurs Haaning
∞
Maren Andersdatter

MAREN KIRSTINE CHRISTENSDATTER I.
døbt 10.-2.-1782 d. 13.-12.-1853
∞ 1.-11.-1816
Jens Laursen Haaning
dødt 28.-9.-1782 d. 14.-4.-1828

Margrethe
f. 3.-6.-1817

MAREN JENSDATTER HAANING II.
f. 25.-4.-1819 d. 6.-6.-1895

∞ 21.-10.-1842
1. Niels Christian Mortensen
f. 1818 d. 5.-6.-1844

∞ 22.-10.-1844
2. Rasmus Chr. Sørensen Sahl
f. 27.-2.-1816 d. 30.-12.-1883

Ane Kirstine Nielsdatter
f. 9.-7.-1843

Niels Kristian Rasmussen Sahl
f. 25.-8.-1845 d. 21.-2.-1918
∞ 25.-7.-1874
Hansine Jensen Nøhr
f. 21.-6.-1856 d. 29.-12.-1941

KAREN MARIE RASMUSSEN SAHL III.
f. 23.-8.-1849 d. 29.-9.-1914
∞ 5.-11.-1867
Niels Pedersen Svenstrup
f. 23.-9.-1839 d. 1.-11.-1920

5 børn

MAREN RASMUSSEN SAHL IV.
BETTE MAREN HAANING
f. 4.-10.-1872 d. 11.-11.-1918
∞ 27.-5.-1893
Søren Hansen

7 børn

In 1832 when the pharmacy opened in Loegstoer, Maren Haaning built a great relationship with them. The pharmacy often got a note from clients with strange words and symbols, so they developed a translation to accommodate the suggestions

I think this is such a fun story, which I didn't know about when I first started in this line of work two decades ago.

Section One

GOOD TO KNOW

Chapter One

HEALTHY MADE SIMPLE

Thousands of years ago, our ancestors lived very differently from what we do today.

Their food was local, in-season food. Their meat was from wild animals, either caught or hunted. That way of living was a perfect match to what our body needs.

Today, we live in a world of a constant hunt for success, and we are all exposed to electronic pollution, sounds, and lights 24/7. We also have many things to balance, with work, kids, family, and friends, but not enough hours in a day!
We don't move as much as our body needs us to, and we've stopped cooking healthy meals for our families. In fact, if you don't make an effort to get organic locally grown food, you often end up getting different additives and fillers which are not good for you. There's more about this in the Mindful Eating section from page 71.

Our busy schedules make us turn to an easy way out, and we tend to cut down on personal time for exercising, fresh air, silence and gratitude. On top of that we start making what I call quick fix choices, such as stocking the pantry with processed food, eating fast food and "take out" because we think it saves time.

This is the fastest and most certain way to disease!

Changing lifestyle and food habits can be quite the challenge. I know, I've been there many times. Just remember, that your current habits have likely been cultivated over many years. I've found that true transformation comes when you focus on changing just 2-3 things at a time. A philosophy I've been sharing with others for two decades.

If you've ever tried a complete lifestyle overhaul, attempting to change fifty things at once, you have most likely also ended up right where you started. The reason is that when you change everything in one go, you'll experience withdrawal symptoms like headaches, cravings, fatigue, restlessness, strong body odor, and irritability. These issues predominantly arise due to two main factors: sugar addiction and detox.

Making changes over time will help your body, mind, and spirit adapt to and appreciate what you are doing. Soon you will be craving healthy habits and you will experience more energy, clear focus, better digestion and sleep.

Chapter Two

THE HUMAN CELL

Our body has about 30 trillion different cells, which all have to communicate smoothly 24/7 to carry out all of our basic functions for survival. We have about 200 different types of cells which include skin cells, fat cells, red blood cells, and nerve cells, and each type has different shapes and weight. It is however, equally important for them all to get the right nutrients in order to maintain optimal function.

This is an illustration of the human cell. It shows you what the different parts of the cell are called, and what they need in order to function 100%. As you can see, it is important we provide the right fuel for the cells, especially when we have more than 30 trillion of them.

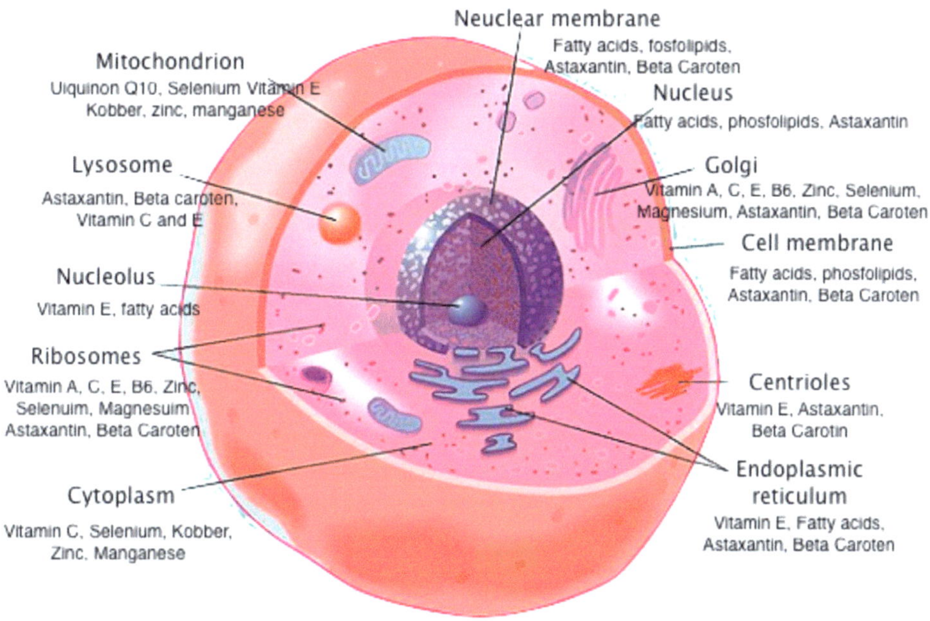

Download full size at www.mygoodwitch.com/bookresources

Cells die every single day and renew as many every single day too. Over time we renew almost all the different cell groups, some more often than others. Most are believed to have a lifespan from 12 weeks to 7 years.

In order to renew our cells for the better, it's very important to feed our body what it needs, so we don't create an environment for cell degeneration and leave worn out cells as a master copy for the new cells. We all know how it looks if we keep copying a copy of a copy, right? It will become unreadable!

The exact same thing happens with our cells. If we keep copying a damaged cell, the new ones will be weak from the beginning. Eventually, this will lead to illness.

Organic whole foods, lots of clean water, quality sleep, exercise, fresh air, silence and gratitude every single day, will help you change the downhill slope and create healthier cells.

Cells Becomes Systems

You now know that you have trillions of cells in your body, and they all belong to different categories. Some of these cell categories are:

Red Blood Cells, Nerve Cells, Muscle Cells, Epithelial Cells, White Blood Cells, Liver Cells, and Pancreatic Beta Cells.

Each category plays different roles in our body. For example, white blood cells are essential for your immune system and nerve cells transmit electrical signals throughout your nervous system.

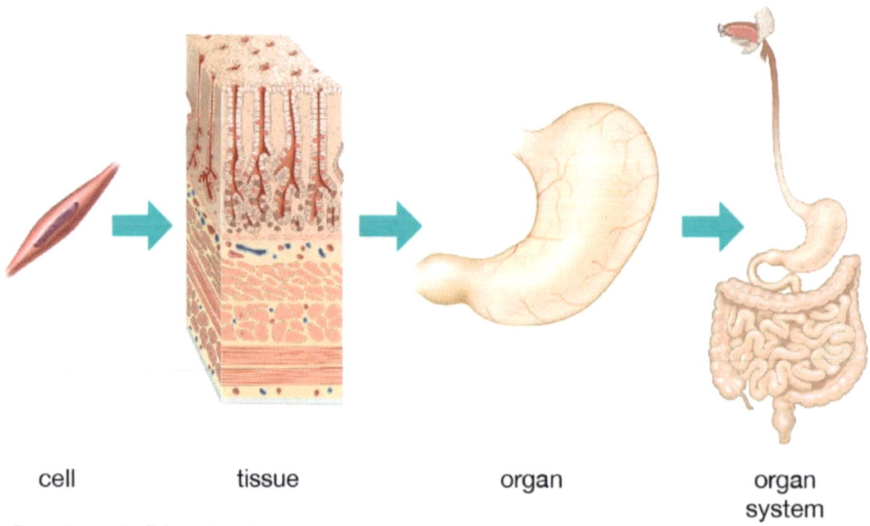

Next, these different cell categories get organized and create tissue. These tissues are:

Muscle Tissue, Connective Tissue and Epithelial Tissue,
which is the skin and lining of the digestive tract.

These different types of tissue then create organs. You have five vital organs:

Heart, Lungs, Liver, Kidneys and Brain and non-vital organs include:
Gallbladder, Pancreas, Stomach, and Intestines.

Last but not least, the organs create body systems. You probably already know all the different systems. However, I think it's important to mention them anyway, as each of these systems plays a vital role in maintaining overall health and functioning.

S***keletal System:*** Consists of bones and cartilage that provide structural support and protection.

Respiratory System: Your lungs and airways that make exchange of oxygen and carbon dioxide happen.

Muscular System: Your muscles enable movement and support body structures.

Cardiovascular System: Includes the heart and blood vessels, and is responsible for circulating blood and delivering oxygen and nutrients to tissues.

Digestive System: Includes organs like the stomach, liver, and intestines; responsible for your digestion and nutrient absorption.

Nervous System: This is the brain, spinal cord, and nerves; these control bodily functions and transmitting signals.

Endocrine System (hormone system): Made up of glands like the pituitary and thyroid that regulate hormones and various bodily functions such as your metabolism and stress response.

Urinary System: Includes the kidneys and bladder that are responsible for filtering and excreting waste products.

Reproductive System: This system is actually a part of the ***Endocrine system***. It is responsible for sexual reproduction and includes organs like the ovaries and testes.

Immune System: Defends the body against infections, vira, and diseases.

Recognizing how cells become tissue, tissue become organs, and organs become systems helps us understand how our body systems work tirelessly to keep us in optimal condition; maintaining balance in it all, from the regulation of hormones to the defense against infections. I hope this helps in understanding the complexity of human biology and the importance of taking care of our health.

Chapter Three

ENERGIES AND RHYTHMS

In Eastern medicine, we are taught how everything in our body is working together to maintain balance and optimal health. Once you get a disease in one system, it will eventually affect other systems. Especially if you don't get to the cause of the problem. All diseases start with cellular inflammation. If we don't find the cause of inflammation, it will become chronic.

Whether it is digestive problems, heart disease, diabetes, arthritis, or autoimmune diseases, *it all starts with inflammation*. This is why it is so important to live by the Seven Steps as mentioned from page 61.

We are created to live in balance with nature - the seasons and the day and night rhythm. Once you understand this natural rhythm, you will be able to take action before an imbalance becomes a disease. You see, it's all about balance between your body, mind, and spirit.

The Main Rhythm

Our body has three main energy cycles in a 24 hour period. It's an energy rhythm where the body has time to clean and create, digest and dispose.

4 am - 12 pm

Time for cleansing and production of enzymes, stomach bile, and hormones, including melatonin. During this phase, the body is focused on detoxification and preparation for the day ahead.

The liver is highly active, breaking down toxins and waste products accumulated overnight. This period is also when the production of melatonin, the hormone responsible for regulating sleep, peaks before gradually declining as the morning progresses.

12 pm - 8 pm

This is when you eat your meals. All your enzymes, stomach bile, and hormones are at their highest level, optimizing digestion. During this period, the body is primed to break down and absorb nutrients from the food you consume.

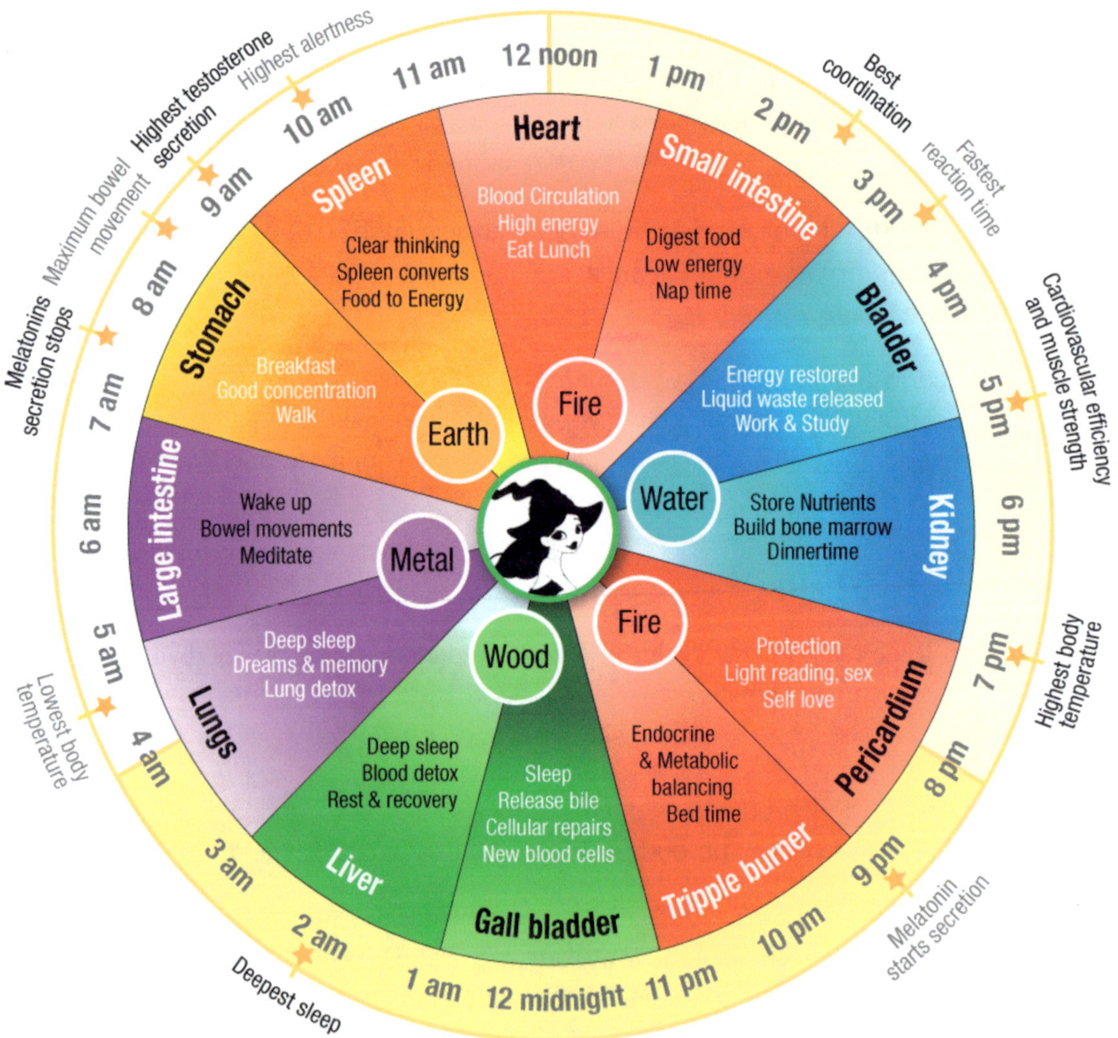
12 noon
1 pm
2 pm
3 pm
4 pm
5 pm
6 pm
7 pm
8 pm
9 pm
10 pm
11 pm
12 midnight
1 am
2 am
3 am
4 am
5 am
6 am
7 am
8 am
9 am
10 am
11 am
Highest alertness
Highest testosterone secretion
Maximum bowel movement
Melatonins secretion stops
Lowest body temperature
Deepest sleep
Melatonin starts secretion
Highest body temperature
Cardiovascular efficiency and muscle strength
Fastest reaction time
Best coordination
Heart
Blood Circulation
High energy
Eat Lunch
Small intestine
Digest food
Low energy
Nap time
Bladder
Energy restored
Liquid waste released
Work & Study
Kidney
Store Nutrients
Build bone marrow
Dinnertime
Pericardium
Protection
Light reading, sex
Self love
Tripple burner
Endocrine
& Metabolic
balancing
Bed time
Gall bladder
Sleep
Release bile
Cellular repairs
New blood cells
Liver
Deep sleep
Blood detox
Rest & recovery
Lungs
Deep sleep
Dreams & memory
Lung detox
Large intestine
Wake up
Bowel movements
Meditate
Stomach
Breakfast
Good concentration
Walk
Spleen
Clear thinking
Spleen converts
Food to Energy
Fire
Water
Fire
Wood
Metal
Earth

Enzymes like amylase, protease, and lipase are secreted in larger quantities, enhancing the digestion of carbohydrates, proteins, and fats respectively. The pancreas and liver work in tandem to ensure efficient digestion and nutrient absorption, providing the energy required for the rest of the day.

8 pm - 4 am

The food you have eaten during the day is turned into energy and stored in your muscles and brain, for you to use within the next 24 hours. This phase is critical for metabolic processes, where the body converts nutrients into glycogen and fat for storage.

Growth hormone levels rise during sleep, facilitating tissue repair and muscle growth.
The brain consolidates memories and processes information gathered throughout the day, enhancing cognitive functions. Additionally, the body undergoes cell regeneration and repair, ensuring that you wake up refreshed and rejuvenated for the next cycle.

The Circadian Rhythm

This rhythm is also known as your biological clock, or biological rhythm. Our different organs have a specific two hour time frame during a 24 hour period, where they have a maximum level of energy, and 12 hours later they have their lowest level of energy.

Let's use the lungs as an example.

The lungs have maximum energy between 3am and 5am. This is where you have your deep sleep and dreams. It is also when your lungs detox. When you are in balance this will happen every night. If you wake up every night within this timeframe 3am and 5am, you most likely have an imbalance in the body system or meridian connected to the lungs.

The illustration on the previous page will help you understand your Bio Rhythm also known as the circadian rhythm. Find it on www.mygoodwitch.com/bookresources

It shows when the different organs are working (have high energy), and why you might have symptoms or issues in the same spot, the same time every day or night. It also shows which Element, from The Law Of The 5 Elements, each organ belongs to.

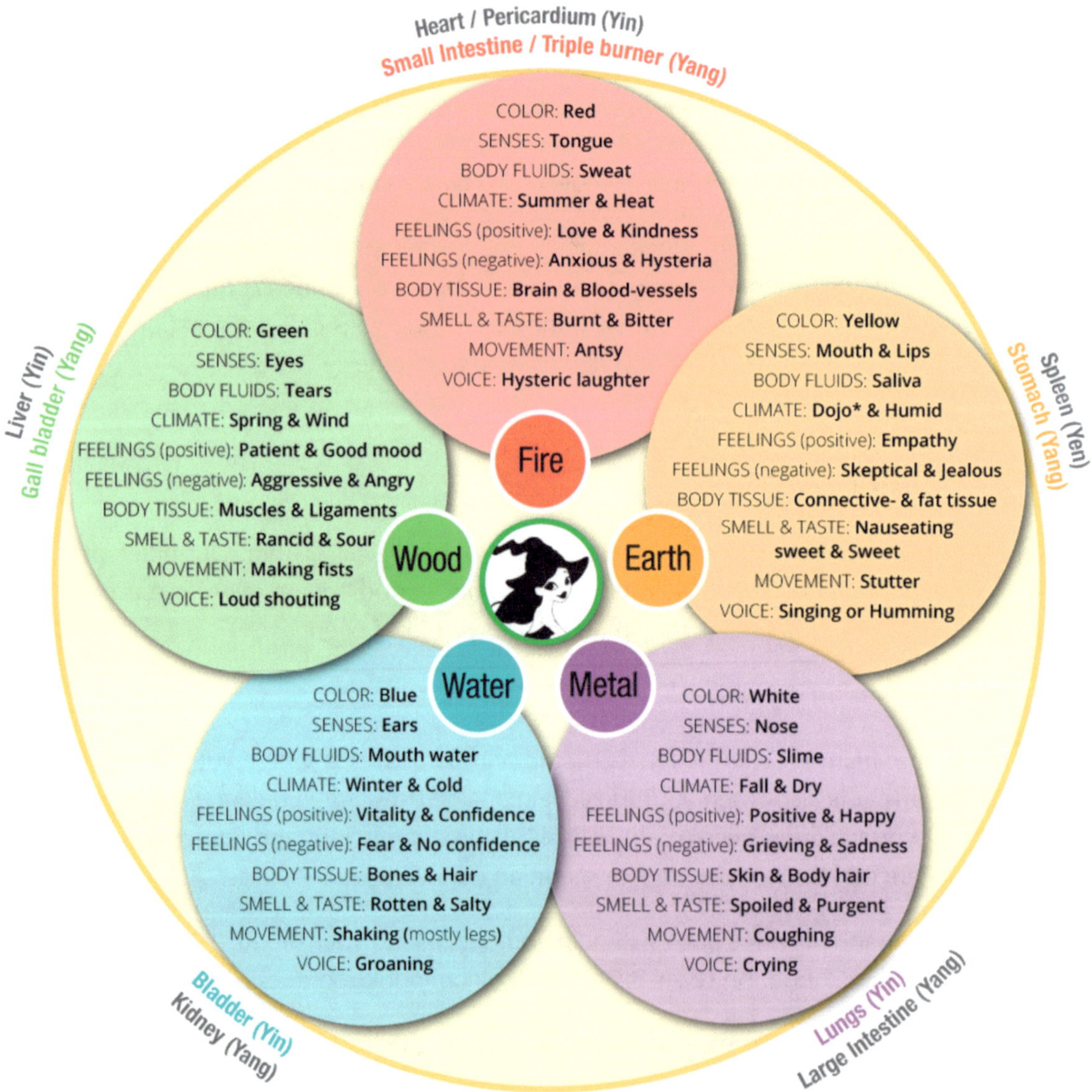

** The shift from one season to the next*

The Law of the 5 Elements

For thousands of years Chinese Medicine has used the bio rhythm as a tool to correct the different imbalances we experience due to incorrect lifestyle. They found a connection between the energies in the sky, the earth, and our body, and named it "The law of the 5 elements".

This theory connects the different elements in nature and the energy between them. The energy flows to and through your body all the time, your entire life, connecting us to these elements of nature.

Wood - Fire - Earth - Metal - Water

The 5 Elements are always changing within you. Some elements become stronger in different seasons both in nature and in life. They always help explain what's going on in the body, as each element has unique characteristics associated with seasons, weather, colors, personality type, imbalances and diseases.

On the previous page I have made an illustration of The 5 Elements, where you can see the different reactions your organs / systems can have when they are out of balance.
You can also find it on www.mygoodwitch.com/bookresources

The 5 Elements are all linked together. Wood feeds Fire, Fire becomes Earth, Earth provides Metal, Metal contains Water, and Water supports Wood. On the other side, Wood roots in Earth, Earth blocks Water, Water puts out Fire, Fire melts Metal, and Metal cuts Wood.

Each element both empowers one another as well as weakens one another. The system is always changing, and striving for balance. Sometimes, one element is dominating within us. This is where our strength lies, but also where we may be most vulnerable.

Harmony among these elements is therefore crucial for your overall well-being. Imbalances can be addressed through acupuncture, reflexology, herbal medicine, dietary adjustments, and the lifestyle changes mentioned in this book.

Wood

A "Wood Personality," is someone who likes being active, muscular, and full of energy. When out of balance they can feel anxious and get easily mad.

Wood personalities might deal with issues like problems with bones or joints, liver imbalances, digestive issues, migraines, or ADD.

Physically, Wood is connected to the liver and gallbladder which means growth and flexibility. A balanced Wood element gives you vitality, energy, strength, and the ability to bounce back.

Mentally, Wood personalities are visionaries, determined and are good at planning. But if things get out of balance it can lead to frustration and anger.

Fire

A "Fire personality" is someone who is passionate, creative, and authoritative. Their body structure may be round in the middle with a pointy top. When out of balance they are often impulsive and irritable.

Fire personalities may suffer from insomnia, high blood pressure, chest pains, headaches, and emotional instability.

Physically, Fire is connected to the heart and small intestine, which means warmth and circulatory functions. A balanced Fire element promotes joy and connection.

Mentally, Fire personalities are charismatic and have a lot of enthusiasm and passion.

Earth

An "Earth personality" is someone who is nurturing, generous, and caregiving. Their body structure is often round and fleshy. When out of balance they tend to be worrying and overthinking.

Earth personalities may suffer from abdominal issues, digestive issues, weight problems, fatigue, or hormonal problems.

Physically, Earth is connected to the spleen and stomach, which means nourishment and stability. A balanced Earth element means proper digestion and absorption.

Mentally, Earth personalities are grounded and nurturing, as well as empathetic and supportive.

Metal

A "Metal personality" is someone who is meticulous, honest, and responsible. Their body structure may be somewhat angular and tall. When out of balance they tend to be melancholy.

Metal personalities may suffer from constipation, lung and skin issues, as well as allergies.

Physically, Metal is connected to the lungs and large intestine, which means purity and clarity. A balanced Metal element means proper respiratory health and elimination.

Mentally, Metal personalities have discipline and are organized, and value structure.

Water

A "Water personality" is someone with an old soul. They are wise, reflective, and private. Their body structures are often puffy and round. When out of balance they tend to be indecisive, fearful, paranoid, and lack willpower.

Water personalities may suffer from back pain, knee pain, reproductive issues, kidney related problems, bladder infections, and hormonal imbalances.

Physically, Water is connected with the kidneys and bladder, which means fluidity and adaptability. A balanced Water element supports the body's filtration and hormonal balance.

Mentally, Water personalities are deep thinkers, have wisdom and self reflection.

Chapter Four

OXIDATIVE STRESS

In our fast-paced world, oxidative stress may seem like yet another fad in the health and wellness world. However, understanding what it is and how it impacts our well-being is crucial for maintaining optimal health. By incorporating organic food choices and embracing mindful living practices, we can take significant steps towards reducing oxidative stress and enhancing our overall quality of life.

What Is Oxidative Stress?

It's a natural process caused by an imbalance between free radicals and antioxidants in the body. Free radicals are unstable molecules with unpaired electrons and act like rust on our cells and genetic material, such as DNA. These free radicals occur during various metabolic processes and diet choices, but can also be triggered by external factors like pollution, EMF, WiFi and UV radiation. Just as rust corrodes the car's metal, free radicals corrode our cells and tissues, causing damage over time. And just like your car, your body needs the right fuel and regular maintenance in order to fight disease.

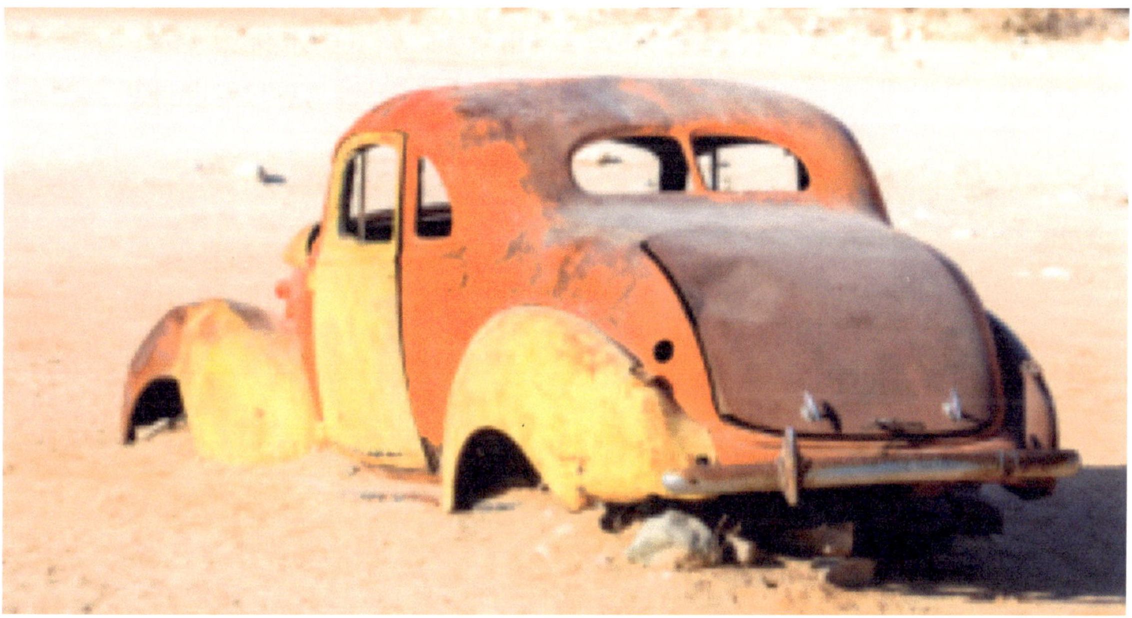

How Does Oxidative Stress Harm Us

Think of oxidative stress as a silent troublemaker messing with your body's inner processes. It's like a city facing some challenges, and your cells are the first ones to feel the effects.
This will lead to a series of issues that affect your health in different ways including those mentioned below.

Cell Damage

Oxidative stress can cause damage to the cells in your body. Imagine your body's cells as a fleet of cars – if these cars get damaged, they won't function properly. Similarly, damaged cells may lead to various health issues.

Aging Process

Picture your body as a well-worn book. Over time, oxidative stress can contribute to the aging process, causing wrinkles, reduced skin elasticity, and other signs of aging. It's like the pages of the book getting crinkled with time.

Inflammation

Oxidative stress can trigger inflammation, which is like a fire breaking out in your city. Inflammation is your body's response to damage, and if it becomes chronic, it may contribute to various diseases.

Disease Connection

Too much oxidative stress is linked to various health problems, such as heart disease, diabetes, and certain types of cancer. It's like a chain reaction – if one part of the city is affected, it can impact the whole system.

Weakening Immune System

Oxidative stress can weaken your immune system, making it harder for your body to fight off infections. It's like having fewer guards in the city, making it easier for troublemakers to cause havoc.

What Can You Do

By adopting a healthy lifestyle and making mindful choices, you can help your body fight oxidative stress and keep it thriving and vibrant.

Making sure to get quality sleep helps the body in its repair and regeneration processes, minimizing cellular damage caused by excess oxidation. Adding mindful practices before bedtime can enhance sleep quality and contribute to a healthier, more balanced state.

Also regular physical activity stimulates the production of antioxidants which act as defenders against oxidative harm.

Mindful eating and living a mindful lifestyle as described in this book, will help reduce oxidative stress. Foods like organic fruits and vegetables are typically packed with antioxidants. These antioxidants play a vital role in neutralizing free radicals and thereby diminishing oxidative stress.

Organic farming practices refrain from using synthetic pesticides and chemicals, which ultimately curtails the intake of harmful toxins associated with oxidative stress. Furthermore, organic foods are known for their nutrient density, offering a rich source of essential vitamins and minerals that bolster the body's antioxidant defense system.

Chapter Five

INFLAMMATION

Inflammation is a natural process that your body uses to protect itself from harm. Think of it as your body's defense mechanism – like a superhero flying in to save the day when there's trouble. However, longtime inflammation will lead to disease.

When your body detects an injury, infection, or any kind of threat, it releases chemicals that cause blood vessels to leak fluid into the tissues. This increased blood flow helps white blood cells reach the affected area and start the healing process. While inflammation is essential for healing, chronic or longtime inflammation is problematic. It can cause damage to healthy tissues as well as arthritis, heart disease, and even certain cancers.

What Causes Inflammation

Inflammation can be triggered by various factors. Consuming high amounts of processed foods, sugars, and unhealthy fats, can promote inflammation in the body.

Chronic stress can lead to inflammation by causing the release of stress hormones like cortisol, which can increase inflammation levels in the body over time.

Exposure to pollutants, pesticides, and other environmental toxins can also trigger inflammation in the body, and persistent infections, such as certain bacterial or viral infections, can cause chronic inflammation if not properly treated. Smoking cigarettes introduces harmful chemicals into the body that can trigger inflammation and damage tissues. Similarly, heavy drinking can lead to inflammation in the body, particularly in the liver and digestive system.

How To Fight Inflammation

Fortunately, there are simple and natural ways to keep most inflammation in check, here are a few:

Mindful eating

As described in the next section from page 75, Mindful Eating is very important.
Having 5 colors on your plate at any meal is not just vibrant and inviting, but it is also rich in antioxidants, which help fight inflammation. Also include sources of omega-3 fatty acids in your diet, such as fatty fish (salmon, mackerel), flaxseeds, and walnuts. These healthy fats have anti-inflammatory properties. And use anti-inflammatory spices when you cook such as turmeric, ginger, garlic, and herbs. Also adding ginger, turmeric, and lemon to your meals can also help fight inflammation. These ingredients are known for their anti-inflammatory properties and can enhance your overall health.

Water is essential

For overall health, including the management of inflammation, you need to drink clean water. It also helps your digestive system excrete toxins and waste. Aim for at least eight glasses a day. Adding lemon to your water as well as drinking ginger tea with lemon, will also help combat inflammation.

Sleep

Lack of sleep can contribute to inflammation. Aim for 7-9 hours of quality sleep each night. Consider creating a relaxing bedtime routine, reducing screen time before bed, and maintaining a consistent sleep schedule. These practices can enhance sleep quality, thereby supporting overall health and reducing the risk of chronic inflammation. Learn more about how to get a good nights sleep in the section about sleep in chapter 8 "My Seven Steps".

Stress-reducing activities

Practicing meditation, deep breathing, or yoga are very beneficial in your fight against inflammation. Also, learn more about how to reduce or eliminate stress in the chapter about Stress management on page .

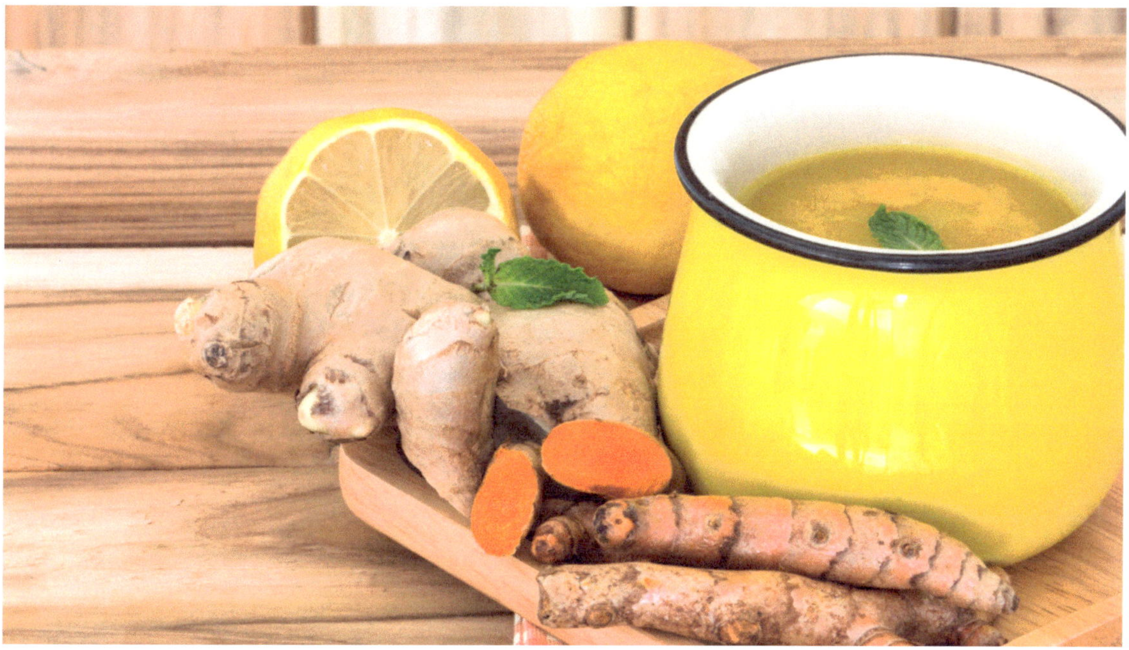

Chapter Six

GUT HEALTH

Around 2000 years ago, the ancient Greek physician Hippocrates stated,

"***All disease begins in the gut.***"

Sadly enough that is still the case!

Our gut is home to trillions of microorganisms, collectively known as the microbiome. These tiny organisms play a crucial role in digestion, nutrient absorption, and even our immune system. About 70% of our immune system is found in our digestive system, so it goes without saying that we have to take good care of it. Medicine, processed and deep fried food, as well as stress are some of today's biggest enemies when it comes to a balanced digestive system.

Therefore, maintaining a healthy balance of gut bacteria is key to preventing inflammation and supporting your overall health.

Incorporate probiotic-rich foods like yogurt (if you tolerate dairy), kefir, sauerkraut, and kimchi into your diet. These foods introduce beneficial bacteria into your gut. Also a quality pre- and probiotic supplement is beneficial to add to your daily supplements. Check my recommendations on www.mygoodwitch.com/bookresources

Including a diet rich in fiber from fruits and vegetables is very beneficial for your gut health. Fiber serves as a prebiotic, and helps the growth of beneficial bacteria in your gut. They also add increased weight, size, and softness of your stool, making a smooth passage of waste through your system. Additionally, fiber adds bulk to your stools and enhances peristaltic movements.

Drink Enough Water

Your digestive fluids, such as saliva and gastric juices, need water to break down food for better digestion and nutrient absorption in the digestive tract.

If you don't drink enough water, it will lead to dehydration, resulting in harder stools and an increased risk of constipation. However, enough water helps soften stools, making them easier to pass through the intestines and preventing constipation. It also reduces the likelihood of experiencing issues like bloating, gas, and discomfort.

Water also plays a vital role in the absorption of nutrients from digested food in the intestines. It helps transport these nutrients through the intestinal walls and into the bloodstream for distribution throughout the body. The mucosal lining of the gastrointestinal tract needs water to maintain its integrity, as well as preventing irritation and inflammation of the lining.

A well-hydrated environment supports the growth and activity of beneficial bacteria in the gut, supporting balanced and diverse microbiota.

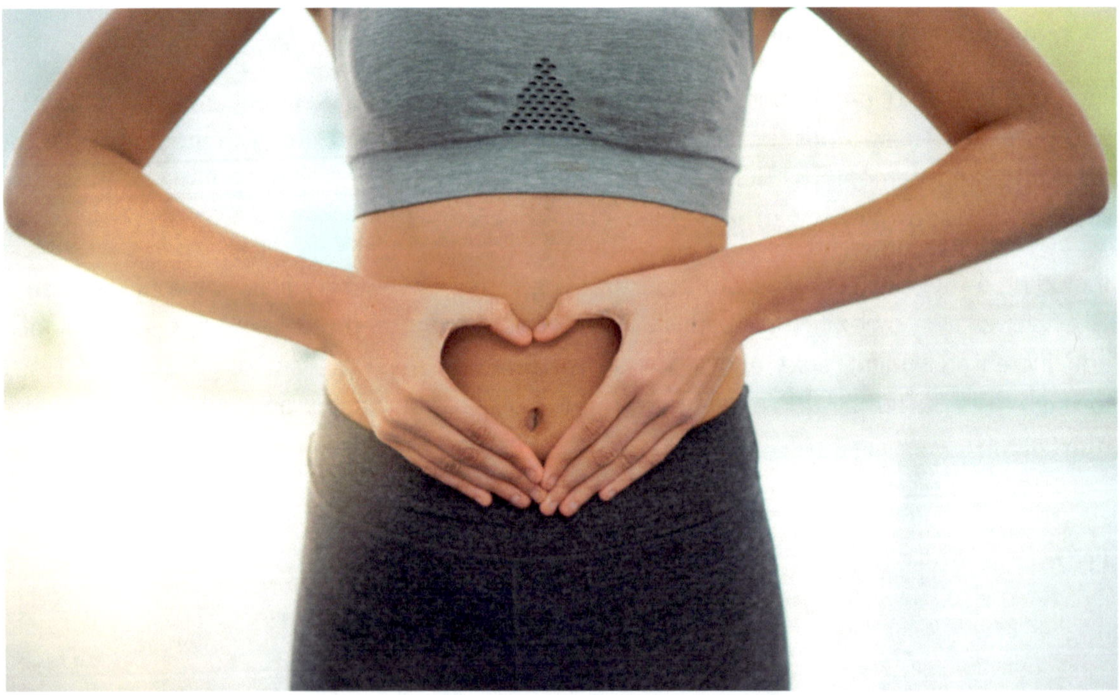

Physical Activity

Regular physical activity is essential for maintaining gut health for several reasons.

Firstly, exercise stimulates the muscles in your gastrointestinal tract, promoting efficient digestion by facilitating the smooth movement of food through your system. This helps prevent constipation and ensures regular bowel movements, which are vital for a healthy gut.

Secondly, physical activity has been shown to positively influence the gut microbiome by increasing the diversity of beneficial bacteria. A diverse microbiome is linked to better overall health and greater resilience against infections and diseases. Exercise encourages the growth of these beneficial bacteria, enhancing gut barrier function and reducing inflammation.

Additionally, exercise helps manage stress levels by triggering the release of endorphins and reducing cortisol, (our stress hormone). Since stress can disrupt the microbiome balance and increase gut permeability, regular physical activity acts as a buffer against these negative effects.

Incorporating activities like walking, jogging, yoga, or any form of movement you enjoy supports not only your cardiovascular and muscular health but also fosters a healthier environment for your gut bacteria. By integrating consistent physical activity into your daily routine, you adopt a holistic approach to enhancing your gut health and overall well-being.

Chapter Seven

PH BALANCE

Maintaining the right pH balance in our body is crucial for overall health and well-being. The human blood pH level should ideally be slightly alkaline ranging between 7.35 and 7.45, and between 6 - 7.50 in urine. However, due to our modern diet and lifestyle, this balance is often disrupted. The easiest way to keep track of your pH Balance is by using a urine pH test, preferably using morning urine.

When our body's pH level is balanced, it creates an environment that promotes proper digestion, efficient nutrient absorption, and effective elimination of toxins. A balanced pH level also helps to support a strong immune system, as harmful bacteria and viruses find it difficult to thrive in an alkaline environment. Additionally, it contributes to improved energy levels, mental clarity, and better overall mood. In other words, by striving for a balanced pH level, we can support our body's natural ability to function optimally and enhance our overall health and well-being.

On the other hand, consuming processed food, fried food, breaded food, and dark meat, as well as indulging in soda, alcohol, energy drinks, tea, and coffee both hot and iced, contributes to an excessive intake of acidic substances.

This overload of acid disrupts the delicate pH balance in our body and creates an environment that is beneficial to the growth of harmful bacteria, viruses, and other pathogens. This will weaken our immune system, making us more susceptible to illnesses and infections. Moreover, an overly acidic environment can also contribute to chronic inflammation.

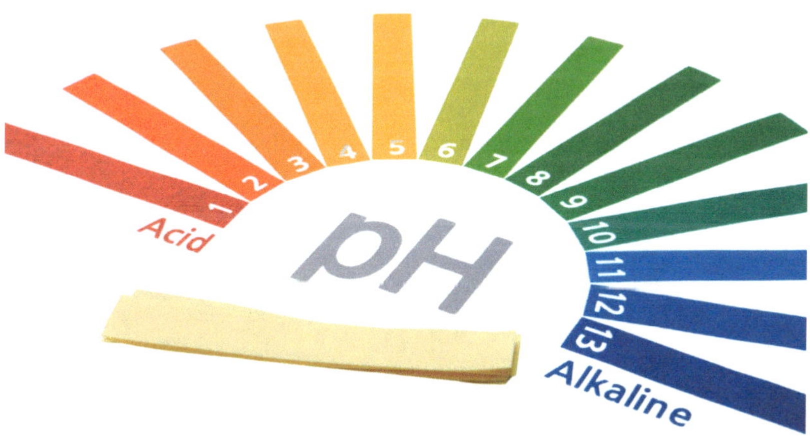

Lets go over some of the most common conditions caused my acid overload:

Inflammation

Excess acidity can lead to chronic inflammation, a condition associated with various diseases, including arthritis, cardiovascular issues, and even cancer. Inflammation is the body's response to injury or harmful stimuli, and a consistently acidic environment may exacerbate this response.

Weakened Immune System

An overly acidic body can compromise the immune system, making it less effective in fighting off infections and illnesses. This vulnerability may increase the risk of frequent colds, flu, and other infections.

Osteoporosis

High acidity levels in the body can lead to the leaching of calcium from bones, contributing to conditions like osteoporosis. The body may pull calcium from bones to neutralize excess acid, resulting in weakened bone structure.

Digestive Disorders

The digestive system requires a balanced pH for optimal function. Excessive acidity may disrupt the balance of digestive enzymes, leading to conditions such as acid reflux, indigestion, and irritable bowel syndrome (IBS).

Weight Gain

Some studies suggest that an acidic environment in the body may be linked to weight gain. Excess acidity could potentially contribute to insulin resistance, making it more challenging for the body to regulate blood sugar and manage weight.

Cancer Growth

While not a direct cause, an acidic environment is believed by some researchers to create a favorable setting for the growth of cancer cells. Maintaining a slightly alkaline pH may be beneficial in reducing the risk of cancer development.

Cardiovascular Issues

Chronic acidity may contribute to cardiovascular problems by promoting inflammation and oxidative stress. Conditions such as high blood pressure and atherosclerosis may be influenced by an imbalanced pH level in the body.

To ensure a more alkaline diet, incorporating certain foods and drinks can be beneficial. Fresh fruits and vegetables, such as leafy greens, cucumbers, broccoli, and citrus fruits, are excellent choices as they are naturally alkaline. Including more plant-based proteins like legumes, nuts, and seeds can also help alkalize the body.

In terms of beverages, consuming herbal teas like chamomile, peppermint, and green tea can provide alkalizing effects. Adding a squeeze of lemon or lime to your water can also boost its alkaline properties. Additionally, incorporating plant-based milk alternatives like almond or coconut milk can be a great way to add alkalinity to your diet.

The Mindful Eating Circle on page 77 can help you change to a more balanced and alkaline diet.

Another tip to consider is to eliminate or reduce the consumption of highly processed and acidic foods. Opt for whole grains, such as quinoa and brown rice, instead of refined grains. Limiting the intake of sugary drinks, processed snacks, and alcohol can also help maintain a more alkaline state.

Lastly, staying hydrated is crucial for maintaining proper pH balance. Drinking enough water throughout the day helps flush out toxins and supports the body's natural detoxification processes. Aim for at least 8 glasses of water per day, and consider adding a pinch of Himalayan salt to your water for added alkalizing minerals.

By being mindful of our food and drink choices, and incorporating more alkaline options into our diet, we can support the body's pH balance and promote optimal health and well-being.

Did you know that it takes 32 glasses of alkaline water (pH 9.5-10) to neutralize one glass of soda?

Chapter Eight

MY SEVEN STEPS

In this chapter, I'll walk you through the basics of each of my "Seven Steps".

It's not just about eating right and exercising, which only make up about 30% of a healthy lifestyle. There are seven areas you need to pay attention to for your overall well-being:

Food, Water, Sleep, Exercise, Fresh Air, Silence and Gratitude.

Think of your body like a puzzle, where each piece is important. Eating healthy and working out are just two pieces of that puzzle. The other five pieces - drinking enough clean water, getting good sleep, breathing fresh air, having moments of silence, and having gratitude - are just as crucial. When all these pieces come together, your body is in balance, or what I like to call being AT-EASE.

If the pieces don't fit together well, you're on the path to DIS-EASE, which means things are out of balance, and you may start feeling unwell. This chapter gives you a quick overview of each of My Seven Steps. As you read the book, you'll dive deeper into why each step is so important for keeping yourself healthy. It's like a roadmap to feeling good and living your best life.

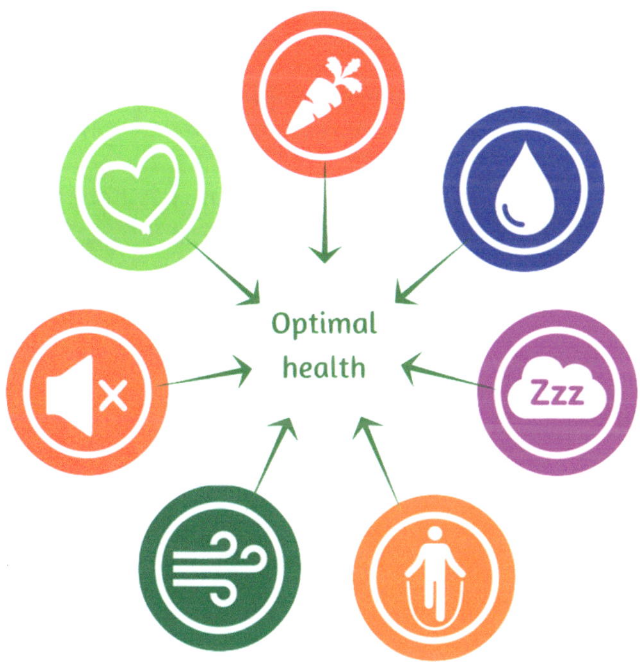

Food

You have to remember we are all unique, and although a diet may work for your friend, it may not work for you! It's not because you're doing something wrong, it's simply because we are not designed to "diet" and leave out important nutrients to lose weight quickly.

Instead we just have to eat clean, organic, and nutrient dense food. Luckily, it's not as complicated as you might think!

When you eat a clean organic diet (meaning, fresh unprocessed food), you avoid the toxins found in most processed foods. These toxins, including artificial colors, flavors, and hidden sugars, accumulate in your body over time, and they are very difficult for the body to excrete. Eat when you are hungry. Eat something from each food group. I usually say to have at least 5 colors on your plate at every meal.

"Eating the Rainbow" will give you all the amazing nutrients found in unprocessed food, and you'll be healthy from the inside out. As a bonus, you will find your natural weight too.

Choose meat from grass fed animals, wild caught fish, eggs from free range chickens, fresh vegetables, nuts, seeds, and natural fats like butter, coconut oil, avocado oil, and vegetable oil.

Of course everything is as organic, locally grown and in season as you can get.

Find more detailed information in Section 2, Mindful Eating.

Water

Water is the most basic and most important substance on the planet, and it makes up 60-70% of our bodies. It is in the air we breathe, and the plants we eat, and it's so vital, that we can only go a few days without it.

The average person doesn't drink enough water, if any water at all. Instead, they substitute other beverages for water, like coffee, sodas, energy drinks and ice teas thinking it's the same thing. I'm sorry to tell you – ***it is not!*** A rule of thumb is, drink half your body weight in ounces each day. A little more when it is hot outside and when you exercise. You can always add herbs, berries, lime, and lemon for taste, if you like.

Clean water has an energizing and cleansing effect that your organs, bones, joints, and digestive system needs for optimal function.

When your body has enough water your system is able to flush out toxins properly instead of storing them in the body where they can cause disease.

Our digestive system needs water for waste to be excreted. With 80% of our immune system being in our digestive system, we really want this to be as healthy as possible!

Also, when your body is dehydrated, it can lead to poor digestive health such as acid reflux, diarrhea, poor nutrient absorption, and constipation.

Sleep

A good night's sleep has a huge impact on our overall health, both physically and mentally. It also gives you more energy and better focus. Yet many do not prioritize their sleep.

Lack of sleep not only affects your immune system, your hormone balance and your cardiovascular system, but also your appetite and stress level! Some of the negative circumstances for a good night's sleep are work pressure, challenges on the home front, and financial instability.

Make sure you're getting enough sleep. Toddlers need 11-13 hours, teenagers 8-10 hours, and adults need an average of 7-9 hours a night!

Go to bed, and get up at the same time every day, including weekends and holidays.

Sleep in a dark, cool and comfortable environment. (You might want to get some extra dark curtains). Eliminate your use of electronic devices at least 1 hour before bedtime.

Relax and substitute the electronics with a good book, soft music or meditation.

Exercise

Exercise plays an important role in your overall mobility and for your organ health, in part by improving your body's circulation of oxygen. Depending on your goals and body type, it's a good idea to incorporate these different types of exercise into your program.

Cardio
improves your heart condition and provides a better blood flow throughout your body.

Strength training
provides stronger bones and more muscles.

Balance training
provides a better reaction-time and coordination.

Breathing exercise
relieves stress and provides oxygen to your cells.

The lymphatic system also depends on movement to excrete toxins and have optimal function. Lymph fluid doesn't circulate like your blood, but is moved forward when your muscles are activated. This is why exercise helps the lymph fluid stay active and flow effortlessly, carrying the white blood cells throughout the body, as well as melting excess fat, and removing bacteria and other harmful materials from your body.

Make it a habit to do some sort of exercise 3-5 times a week, for at least 30 minutes.

Fresh Air

Make it a daily priority to get fresh air, whether rain or shine. Spend at least 30 minutes each day taking a walk, going for a run, a bike ride, or whatever you like to do outside. The benefits of this routine are numerous. Fresh air infuses your cells with vital oxygen, rejuvenating your body and filling up your energy levels. Also, it boosts serotonin production, the hormone responsible for your mood and overall well-being. Furthermore, fresh air is renowned for its positive effects on your immune system and digestion, as well as sharpening your focus and promoting mental clarity.

Remember: There is no such thing as bad weather, only wrong clothing!

Grounding

Our modern lifestyle can lead to a build up of positive ions in our bodies over time, which results in different health issues such as fatigue, anxiety, pain, sleep disorders, and cardiovascular problems. Fortunately, the Earth is rich in negative ions, offering a natural solution to restore balance and well-being through the practice of grounding.

To reconnect with nature, simply make it a habit to step outside barefoot each morning, whether on the ground, grass, or gravel. You can walk around or just sit in silence and become one with nature. Start with just 5 minutes and gradually increase your daily grounding time to 30 minutes or more.

Silence

Silence is another important part of your well-being. Take a break when it fits into your daily routine. Whether you like to meditate or listen to quiet music is entirely up to you – as long as you find the kind of silence that works best for you.

Experiencing silence through meditation will boost your self-esteem, motivation and joy. It gives you mental strength and brings you in contact with your inner self and back to the present.

Make sure to have at least 15 minutes of silence twice a day. If you are just starting, do 5 minutes twice a day, and work your way up.

Prepare your brain and body for silence by doing 5 deep breaths before you start.

Silence helps you reflect on what has happened, recharge your batteries, and to relax, by freeing your mind from the constant stream of noise and stimuli that surrounds you at all times.

The physiological benefits of silence include lower blood pressure, a boosted immune system, and reduced stress. Leave your cell phone, computer and other electronic devices alone during all meals, and be present with people around you. You'll be amazed at the benefits it will bring you and your loved ones.

Silence also helps you to be creative, realize your dreams, as well as discover who you are and how you feel!

Gratitude

Gratitude is without a doubt one of the most overlooked tools we have access to every day. It doesn't cost anything, doesn't take much time, yet the benefits are enormous!

In today's world, it is so easy to be caught up in a negative thought process, where fear, frustration, and condemnation often takes over. This state of mind can lead to depression and melancholy, which is certainly not good for your health.

When practicing gratitude however, you will experience a positive impact on your health, both physically and mentally. It also gives you more empathy for others, increases your self-esteem and helps you value other people's achievements. Additionally, it will help you reduce stress, anxiety as well as, support a good night's sleep.

Make it a habit and write at least 5 things you are grateful for every single night before going to bed. It will make a big difference in your path to optimal health and balance.

Have an "attitude of gratitude"
to create a positive balance in your mind and your life.

To create a good foundation for your health,
your cells need whole food
packed with all the essential nutrients.

You also need to drink enough water,
a good nights sleep, get fresh air, exercise, have silence and
gratitude every single day to maintain life!

~Birgitte Haaning Christensen

Section Two

MINDFUL EATING

Chapter Nine

A BALANCED DIET

Our Food

It is nice to eat out once in a while, but I do not like the taste I get from trans-fat, because most resturant kitchens cooks with cheap vegetable oil. This type of trans-fat creates free radicals and oxidative stress in our body. More about the different types of fats and oils later. Anyway, oftentimes when we talk about going out, we end up eating at home!

I really enjoy cooking our own meals. And I really like to take out a day to prepare some easy meals for a busy day! In this chapter I will share exactly what mindful eating means. And, I will teach you just how simple a healthy lifestyle can be.

We don't count calories and we don't leave out any of the food categories.

Your body is not a simple math problem where you can just add and subtract calories. It is way more complex than that. You need a variety of nutrients like vitamins, minerals, proteins, fats, and carbs in order for everything to work properly. (Remember the Human Cell illustration on page 21?). Although it is very popular to count calories, that is NOT the way to do it. When you focus only on how many calories you get, you miss out on whether you're getting the right nutrients your body needs. It's like obsessing over the number of puzzle pieces without caring if they actually make a complete and healthy picture. Plus, not all calories are created equal. A hundred calories of broccoli and a hundred calories of chocolate don't do the same things in your body. The quality of what you eat matters more than just the quantity.

I do agree that some of the different diets out there can be a good kickstart in changing your eating habits, However, NONE of them (not even vegetarian and vegan), are good for you in the long run. You need nutrients from **ALL** the food groups.

"It is not necessarily fat, protein and carbohydrates that makes you fat, it is the quality of them"

~Dr. Mark Hyman

You Can Eat Almost Anything

I have a couple of sayings I like to share with clients to make it easier to remember what healthy food is, and what to choose when grocery shopping.

"If the food has been able to grow, run, fly, or swim on its own, you can eat it"

"Buy organic, in season and locally grown food after the "farm to table" principal which equals shorter transport and not processed"

"If you buy processed food, go for five or less ingredients"

"Always shop the outer perimeter of the grocery store"

When you switch out the food that makes you store fat, crave sugar and "bad" carbs, with food that nourishes you, it will help you stay on course and help avoid any type of withdrawal.

You will learn how to stop eating fattening, processed, empty calories, and starchy foods, and how to eat colorful, nourishing, and healthy foods. What is more inviting than a plate full of colors?

You will also learn how to avoid consuming unhealthy, high-calorie, processed foods as well as starchy options, and how to embrace a vibrant and nourishing diet, filled with colorful and nutritious foods. As a result, you will see a positive change in your mood, your energy, your sleep, and your overall well-being almost immediately.

Many years ago, a good friend and great mentor of mine from Denmark, Frede Damgaard, taught me the importance of how we should divide our food intake for a day, and two decades later, we still live as close to this as possible. It doesn't mean we never eat something we know is not good for us. When we do we allow ourselves to enjoy it and then we are back on track the next day.

Remember this is a journey, and sometimes you will hit obstacles. The important thing is how fast you get back up.

The Mindful Eating Circle

Using this Mindful Eating circle, let's take a look at how your daily food consumption should look. Please bear in mind these are just some of the foods in the different categories.

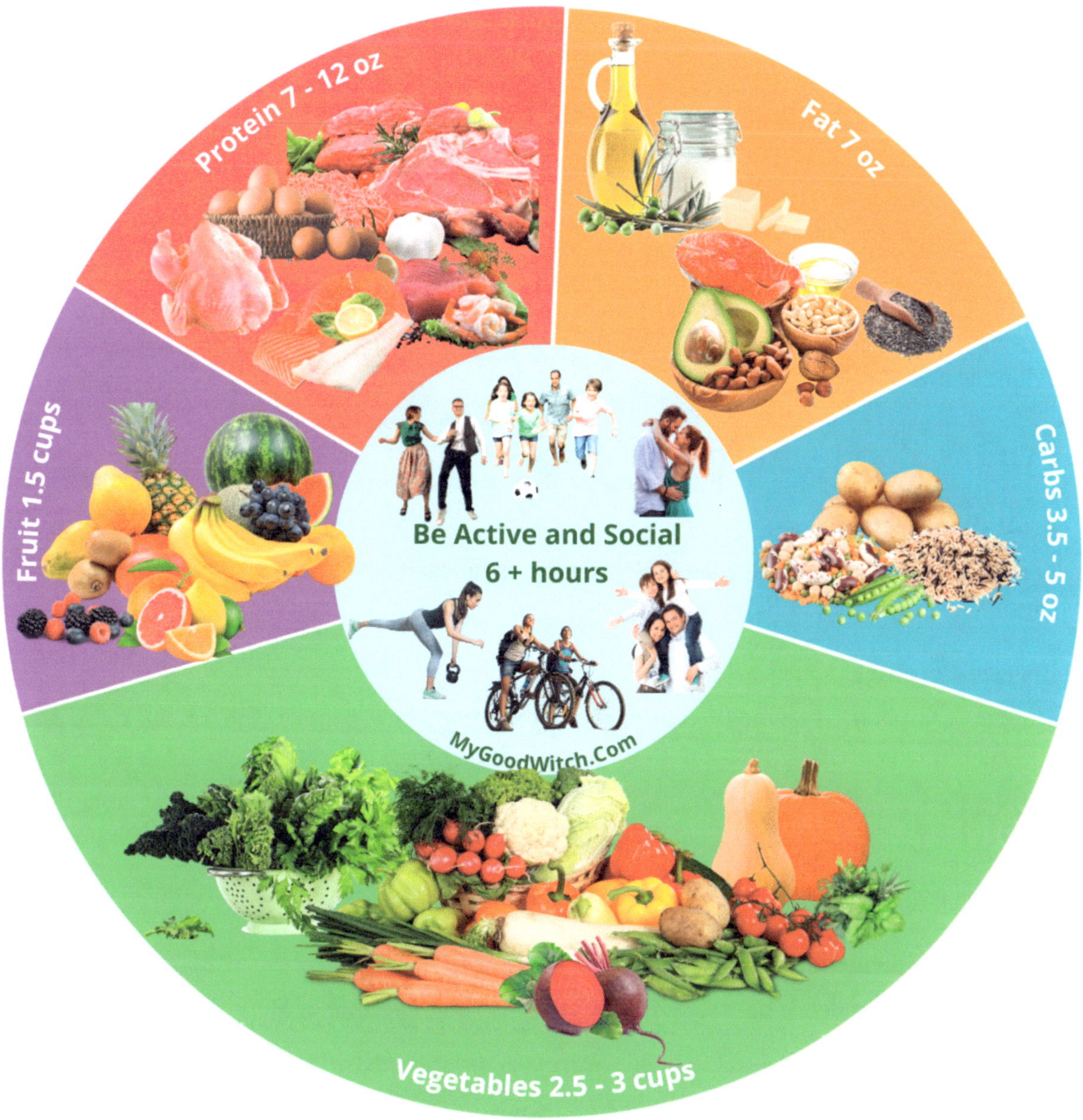

Protein 7 - 12 oz
Fat 7 oz
Carbs 3.5 - 5 oz
Vegetables 2.5 - 3 cups
Fruit 1.5 cups
Be Active and Social
6 + hours
MyGoodWitch.Com

Vegetables - 2 ½ - 3 cups

These can be raw, boiled, baked, sautéed, broiled, and grilled.

Leafy greens and cabbage - 1 1/4 cup

Such as spinach, bitter lettuce, leeks, peas, squash, celery, all types of kale, cabbage, red cabbage, brussels sprouts, pointed cabbage, cauliflower, and broccoli.

Root fruits - ¾ - 1 cup

Such as carrots, parsnips, beets, radish, celery root, all types of onion, potatoes, and sweet potatoes.

Other vegetables - ½ cup

Such as garlic, chili, asparagus, fennel, cucumber, peppers, tomatoes.

All types of herbs, spices, sprouts, and microgreens. Also ginger, turmeric, and horseradish belong in this category.

Fruit & Berry - 1 cup

Fruit - ¾ cup

Apple, pear, banana, peach, pineapple, pomegranate seeds, grapefruit, kiwi, grapes, orange, lemon, lime, mandarin, plums, and melons.

Berries - ½ cup

Blueberry, raspberry, strawberry, blackberry, gooseberry, black currant, apricot, fig, date, goji, and acai.

Protein - 7 - 12 oz

This can be boiled, baked, grilled or broiled, and in some cases raw.

Seafood - wild caught only

Salmon, cod, flounder, tuna, snapper, mackerel, herring, grouper, mahi mahi, squid, lobster, clams, oysters, and mussels.

Animal meat - organic grass-fed and free range

Veal, lamb, game, beef, pork, and poultry like chicken, duck, turkey, pheasant, and quail.

Plant based - Beans, lentils, legumes, peas, chickpeas.

The fibers in these are very strong which makes them difficult for your digestive system to break down. Only eat this group once a week.

Healthy Fats - 1 - 1 ¼ cup

Make sure to get a ⅓ from each group, saturated, polyunsaturated, and monounsaturated fats. (All vegetable oils should be organic cold pressed virgin oils).

Plant based - ¾ cup

Coconut-, Olive-, Avocado-, almond- flax seed- and sunflower oil.
Almonds, pecans, walnuts, cashews, and macadamia nuts. Sunflower-, pumpkin-, chia-, hemp-, flax- and sesame seeds. Avocado and homemade nut butters

Animal based - ¼ - ½ cup

Butter from grass-fed free range animals. Fish and fish oil supplements including astaxanthin.

Carbs (starches) - ½ - ¾ cup

Wild rice, quinoa, oat, barley, and ray. Potatoes, beans, legumes, and lentils.

Cooling starchy foods like potatoes after cooking triggers the formation of resistant starch, similar to fiber, offering health benefits like improved gut health and blood sugar control. Additionally, it lowers their glycemic index, leading to more stable energy levels. Resistant starch reduces caloric density, aiding in weight management, and enhances flavor and texture, making dishes more enjoyable.

Also, soaking rice, beans, and lentils cuts cooking time, improves digestibility by breaking down complex sugars and proteins, reduces phytic acid content, and enhances mineral absorption as well as texture and flavor.

" The food you eat can be either the safest and most powerful form of medicine, or the slowest form of poison"

~Ann Wigmore, founder of the Hippocrates Health Institute

The Key Is Fiber

It is probably not news to you that you should eat more fibers. But do you know what fibers are, and why they are so essential for your gut health?

Hippocrates said more than 2000 years ago -

"All disease starts in the gut"

This couldn't be more true, and yet so many people of this day and age still do NOT have a healthy gut. Let's change that together!

There are 2 types of fibers, soluble and insoluble, and they both play an important part when it comes to optimal health.

Soluble fibers

Soluble fiber is found in oat bran, barley, nuts, seeds, beans, lentils, peas, and some fruits and vegetables. It is also found in psyllium, just which is a common fiber supplement.
These fibers absorb the water in your stool, and form a soft gel like substance, making it easier to pass. They also help promote your bowel movement and regularity.

Insoluble fibers

Insoluble fibers are found in wheat bran, vegetables and whole grains. These do not dissolve in water. They travel through the intestines completely intact, and help a faster elimination of stool and toxins. Insoluble fibers also add bulk to the stool, which help lower the risk of disease.

Benefits Of Fiber

Fibers are mainly found in vegetables, fruits, legumes, and whole grains, and have several health benefits. They play an important role in your gut health by supporting your bowel movements and your gut microbiota. They help prevent digestive issues and chronic health issues. Fibers are not broken down by your body, like carbs, fat, and protein. Instead, they pass relatively intact through your stomach, small intestine, and colon and are finally transported out of your body.

The good thing is, because fibers are not broken down, they are great detoxifiers of toxins and other waste materials.

Consuming a diet high in fiber, you'll help your digestive system increase the weight, size, and softness of your stool so you are able to move any waste smoothly through the system. You also decrease the chances of constipation, as well as too loose and watery stool. When it comes to detox, fibers play an important role too. Toxins build up in our colon where they stick to the intestine wall. This build up stops nutrients from being absorbed, which will lead to disease. When eating a diet high in fibers, you help eliminate these build ups, and transport them out.

Studies show that consuming a diet rich in both soluble and insoluble fibers not only contributes to weight management but also decreases the risk of various health issues such as diverticulitis, hemorrhoids, diabetes, and heart disease. Additionally, it aids in maintaining balanced cholesterol levels, lowering the risk of colon cancer, and supporting weight reduction or maintenance.

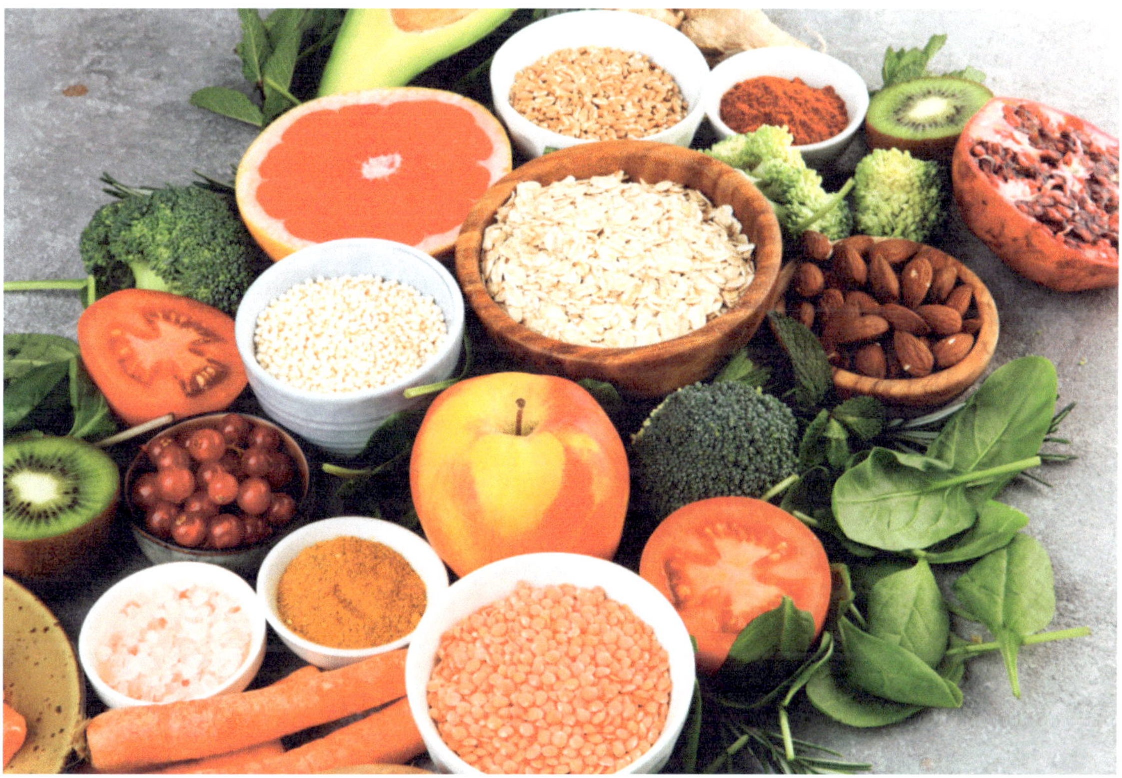

Go back to The Mindful Eating Circle, and see just how much vegetables, fruit, legumes, and grain you should eat every day. If you feel like you need a little extra you can buy some Psyllium Husk capsules to support your fiber intake. Just remember to increase slowly, and drink plenty of water, as you don't want to create constipation when you are not used to fiber.

A little side note:
I'm not sure you can get too much fiber. But, some say that too much fiber may cause bloating, gas, and pain. If that is the case, try to drink more water before cutting down on your fibers.

Carbohydrates

Carbohydrates, or carbs, is something many diets focus on and tell you to avoid. I totally disagree! You are not supposed to count calories or carbs. You need carbs in your diet. However, not all carbs are good carbs, so let me break down the different types of carbs.

There are 3 main groups of carbohydrates

Fibers

This is a complex carb, and your body can't break down most fibers. This is a good thing because the fibers will help you feel full and prevent overeating. Fibers also help prevent digestive problems like constipation, help lower cholesterol, and help regulate your blood sugar, which we touched on earlier. Great sources of fiber are from vegetables, fruits, beans, nuts, seeds, and grains.

Sugars

This is a simple carbohydrate because they are the most basic form of carbs. Sugar is often added in processed foods, desserts, breakfasts, candy, and soda and other drinks. Please keep in mind that refined sugar is NOT a natural source of sugar. More about that later. Sources of natural sugar are mainly found in fruits, vegetables, and dairy.

Starches

These are also complex carbohydrates and are basically made from simple sugars strung together. In order for starches to be used in our body, it needs to be broken down into sugar, so we can use it as energy. When that energy is not used, it's stored as fat. Starch is found in processed products like pasta, bread, cereal, and fat free products. Natural sources of starches are found in root fruits, potatoes, peas, legumes, and corn. See The Mindful Eating Circle on page 77.

Processed Food

In most processed foods, you will find added sugar or fructose. The food industry adds these intentionally in order to trick your brain to eat more, and keep you in the sugar addiction.

The more sugar you eat, the more sugar you will crave - meaning you'll buy more of their products.

Other things like artificial color, flavor, and sweetener as well as added nitrate, different types of gums, and preservatives are found in processed food. You really want to avoid all these.

Just because you buy organic, gluten free or vegan, doesn't mean it is healthy - you still have to watch out for all the fillers in processed food items. That's why I want you to buy fresh whole food, and prepare your own meals!

Meal prepping

When you meal prep a couple times a week, you are more likely to stay true to your new healthy lifestyle when it comes to food choices. Try to have a written meal plan for the week. Make bigger batches of dinner and either freeze or store in glass containers. That gives you easy access to nutritious food on a busy day. You also avoid all the additives and sugars found in most packaged and processed products.

Here are some of the things I do to prepare meals for an easier and healthier week.

- Everything is stored in mason jars or other glass containers.
- Prepare fruit and veggies for juicing
- Making a huge bowl of salad, or Grab 'n Go salad jars.
- Cook a whole bag of wild rice, and freeze in smaller portions
- Make hummus. For a colorful version, you can make pea- or beet hummus.
- Prepare meat of your choice, and store either in the fridge for use the next couple days, or freeze it for a busy or lazy night.
- Cook a bag of potatoes either boiled or grilled, and store in glasses. You also prepare hash browns and mashed potatoes.

These are just some of the things I prepare. I also have our paleo bread, crackers, and breakfast crunch ready for the week.

Find inspiration on www.mygoodwitch.com/recipes/

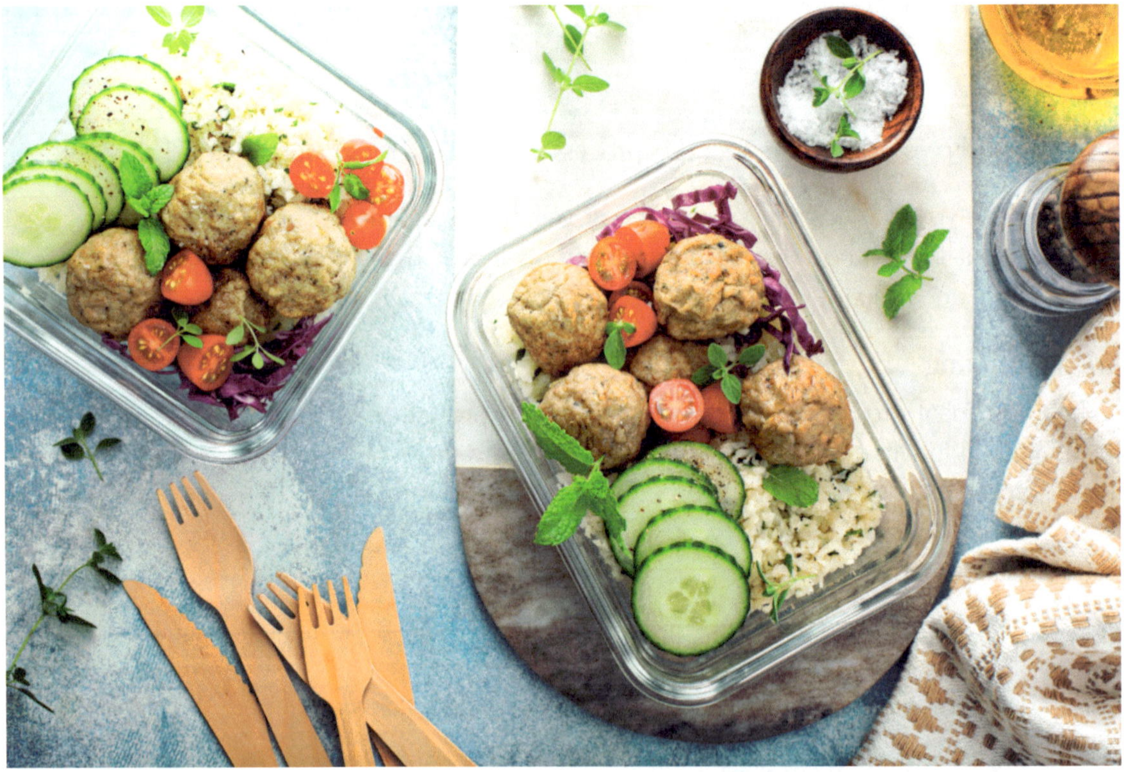

When we grill a whole chicken, I make a very simple broth of the carcass. Put the carcass in your slow cooker and fill it with water. Let it simmer overnight. In the morning, strain the broth through a cheesecloth into wide mouth mason jars, and store it in your freezer. It makes it easy when you want to make soups, stews, and casseroles. I prefer not to add any vegetables or spices until I use the broth later on.

Reboot Your Sugar Intake

A thing you might not know about sugar is the fact that it is extremely addictive. Some experts even say it is more addictive than heroin, which to me, is very scary, but unfortunately very true. Sugary drinks like sodas, iced tea, energy drinks and sports drinks, are extremely high in sugars. Even the zero sugar versions. Candy, baked goods, cereal, yogurt, plant milk, and ice cream also have a high amount of added sugar.

And last but not least, the group of food we wouldn't think contained sugar are ketchup, tomato sauce, dressings, protein bars, bacon, and chicken. Almost all types of processed foods contain one or more different types of sugar. If you don't believe me - take a look in your pantry and read the labels.

You might not recognize that it is sugar because it has many different names.

Look out for all types of syrup (best known is corn syrup and high fructose corn syrup), but also cane juice, agave nectar, and palm sugar, as well as the supposedly "healthy" types of sugar like beet sugar and processed stevia.

No matter what it's called, sugar is sugar, and in excess, it will affect your body negatively in many ways. You may not feel it today or tomorrow, but over time you will create disease.

Below is a typical American daily diet that does not even include the really "bad" options.

Breakfast

Cereal, granola, bread, doughnuts, and other baked goods

Lunch

Sandwich, pizza, pasta or any Fast Food choices, including lunch restaurants.

Dinner

Pasta, rice, mac 'n cheese, pizza, any dishes with cheese, and any Fast Food choices.

Then add the different types of drinks you consume in a day! The daily sugar intake adds up really quickly. If you can recognize this, you get way too much sugar and trans-fat, and are well on your way to disease. A lifestyle change is needed if you want to reverse or avoid disease.

Why Is Sugar So Addictive

The reason why sugar is so addictive is because it stimulates the "pleasure" center in your brain, by producing dopamine.

Dopamine is a neurotransmitter which acts like a hormone, and plays an important role in many body functions such as memory, movement, motivation, mood, and attention.

The first time we are introduced to the taste "sweet", is when we are breastfed for the first time. The dopamine release makes you feel happy, safe, and comfortable while in your mothers arms. This memory is stored in your brain, and you will always remember it, which is one of the reasons why we easily get addicted to sugar.

Unfortunately, the food industry is using this positive memory as a trigger to get us hooked on their processed food. I am not here to tell you that you can't have sugar; I am here to tell you why you should cut your sugar intake down to a minimum.

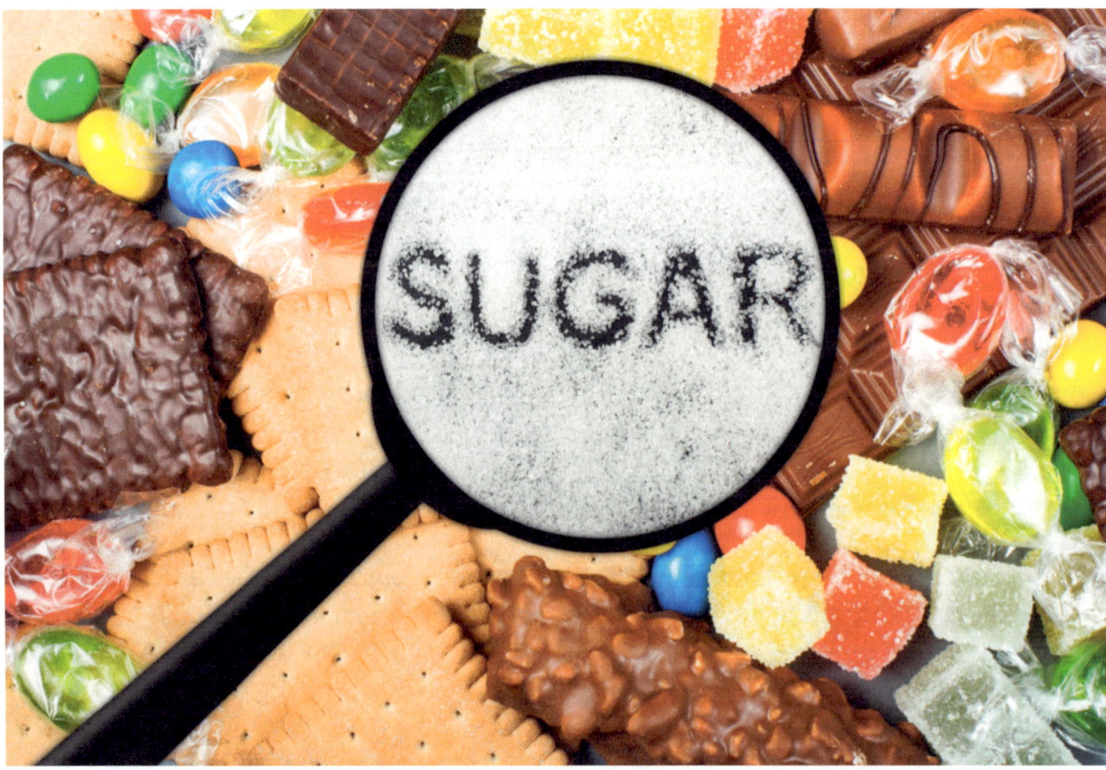

For decades we have been told to eat zero sugar, low-fat, and zero fat. ***That is NOT natural. You need some sugar and you need a lot of fat***. When natural fat is taken out of let's say yogurt, something else is added. Usually this something is different types of processed sugars and starches. This is a very bad combination. Your body converts all the extra starch into sugar and it is used as energy. However, so is all the extra sugar. When this extra sugar is not used, due to lack of exercise and movement, the only way the body can deal with it, is to turn it into fat, and store it in your tissue.

That is just one more reason why you should eat food as nature designed it, and not how mankind has manipulated it. Your body struggles to recognize these hybrid sources of food, as well as too much food grown outside your area.

Eat organic, in season, and locally grown

When you teach your body to work on less sugar and learn your way around the food jungle, you will be able to feel just how much sugar you can handle, without falling back into the addiction. You will also quickly learn how to fuel your body the right way and keep a steady blood sugar level throughout the day.

The Different Types Of Sugar

The four different groups of sugar

Glucose - food sugar
Fructose - fruit sugar
Sucrose - table sugar
Lactose - dairy sugar

And, let's not forget the carbohydrates. Remember from earlier, every carb that's not a fiber, goes through the same breakdown process as sugar, and is therefore also stored as fat when it's not used.

Glucose

This is the main sugar found in your blood. Along with fat, glucose is your main source of energy. It is the simplest carbohydrate, and you get it from the food you eat, such as vegetables, fruit, nuts and grain. When you eat, your body starts working to process glucose.

Enzymes start this breakdown process with help from the pancreas. The pancreas, which produces hormones including insulin, is a very important part of how your body deals with glucose. When you eat, your body signals the pancreas that it needs to release insulin to deal with the rising blood sugar level.

Fructose

Fructose is naturally found in fruits and vegetables where it occurs in a relatively low amount. It needs to be converted into glucose by your liver, before it can be used as energy.

Unfortunately, fructose is now used to make processed sugars like high fructose corn syrup and agave syrup. In fact, if you see added sugar on a label it is most likely from one of these unnatural types of fructose.

Because this unnatural fructose is added to most processed foods, you consume an excessive amount every day, without knowing it. This will cause major metabolic disorders, which may lead to weight gain, visceral fat, insulin resistance, high blood pressure, high cholesterol, and fatty liver. Although fructose usually is found in low amounts in vegetables and fruit, most people think dried fruit and fresh made juice is healthy. Here is why they are NOT!

Dried fruit

When water is removed from fruit, the sugar gets very concentrated.

Even if you buy it organic and free from additives, the dried fruit has the same amount of sugar as the fresh fruit. Problem is, without the water naturally occurring in fruit, you don't get the same feeling of being full. This typically results in eating a larger amount of dried fruit, as you would fresh food - meaning you get more sugar. I would still recommend dried fruit over candy any time.

Fresh juice

Juicing has become very popular over the last decades, and we have been led to believe that we can get the daily recommendation of fruit and vegetables by juicing. THIS IS NOT TRUE! You miss one big factor - the fiber.

When you remove the fiber from your fruit and vegetables, you have isolated fructose, leading to a spike in your blood sugar and increased insulin production. This over-consumption of fructose can oftentimes lead to weight gain and increased risk of type 2 diabetes.

However, if you make sure to get a solid meal rich in fibers with your fresh pressed juice, you should be good. And don't throw away the pulp. I make pizza crust and small flat breads of pulp, and it is delicious. That way you get more fibers in, and there is no waste.
Find my recipe on www.mygoodwitch.com/recipes

Sucrose

Naturally found in vegetables, fruits, and nuts. Sucrose is, when digested, broken down into glucose and fructose, where the glucose is picked up by your blood cells supported by insulin and is used for energy. The fructose is handled by the liver, and does not need insulin.

Sucrose, mostly from sugar cane and sugar beets, is known as table sugar and is found as added sugar in most processed and packaged foods and drinks. The excessive consumption of un-natural sucrose is linked to obesity, type 2 diabetes and heart disease.

Lactose

Lactose is naturally found in milk from cows and goats and humans. Because lactose is a critical nutrient in breast milk for infants, you are able to produce lactase, which breaks down the lactose. Infancy is the stage in life where this production of lactase is highest. Production drops quickly after weaning, and typically diminishes as you age. However, if you are like most people, you still get a lot of dairy products every day. You may even have an intolerance without knowing it. Lactose intolerance is known to cause bloating, cramps, diarrhea, and gas. We'll talk more about this later.

What Does Sugar Actually Do To Your Body

We now know why we should stay away from sugar and processed food. But what does sugar actually do to us?

Your Brain

Eating sugar gives your brain a huge surge of a feel-good chemical called dopamine. That explains why you're more likely to crave a candy bar at 3 p.m. than an apple or a carrot. Because whole foods like fruits and veggies don't cause the brain to release as much dopamine, your brain starts to need more and more sugar to get that same feeling of pleasure. This causes the "gotta-have-it" feeling for your after-dinner ice cream that is so hard to shake.

Your Pancreas

When you eat, your pancreas pumps out insulin. But if you're eating way too much sugar and your body stops responding properly to insulin, your pancreas starts pumping out even more insulin. Eventually, your overworked pancreas will break down and your blood sugar levels will rise, setting you up for type 2 diabetes and heart disease.

Your Liver

An abundance of added sugar usually contains fructose or high fructose corn syrup. Fructose is processed in the liver. Large amounts of fructose can damage the liver.

When excessive amounts of fructose is broken down in the liver, and not used as energy, it transforms into fat and can over time cause:

- Non-alcoholic fatty liver disease (NAFLD): This is seen as excess fat build-up in the liver.
- Non-alcoholic steatohepatitis (NASH): is a fatty liver, inflammation and "steatosis," which is scarring of the liver. Scarring eventually cuts off blood supply to the liver. Many of these develop into cirrhosis and one will eventually need a liver transplant.

Your Skin

Another side effect of inflammation is that it makes your skin age faster.

Excess sugar attaches to proteins in your bloodstream and creates harmful molecules called "AGEs," (advanced glycation end products). These molecules do exactly what they sound like they do: age your skin. They have been shown to damage collagen and elastin in your skin protein fibers that keep your skin firm and youthful. The result? wrinkles and saggy skin.

Dairy

I am sorry to have to tell you but dairy products are to be avoided all together. As I mentioned earlier, we are NOT designed to drink milk all our life. We are ONLY supposed to have milk when we are breastfed as infants, because we simply can't break down lactose and casein after weaning. That is why most people can't metabolize lactose, as well as casein, which is one of the toughest protein sources to break down.

In fact about 70% of all people are not able to digest dairy, and actually have a sensitivity or an intolerance, without knowing it. This will cause stress and inflammation, which will affect your immune system. Casein can create neuropeptides and affect the brain in the same way as heroin.

According to Dr. Lipman, sensitivity to casein can cause:

excess mucus production, respiratory problems,
constipation, gas, bloating and/or diarrhea.

Dairy sensitivity and intolerance in general, is also known to cause:

skin issues like acne, rashes, redness, eczema, as well as autoimmune diseases,
inflammation and irritable bowel syndrome (IBS).

The casein content in cheese is higher than in milk, which is why you can easily feel like you crave cheese. This means you actually have a cheese addiction, just like you can have a sugar addiction.

Think about it for a minute - Have you ever had a cheese heavy meal at night, waking up the next morning with a stuffy nose, slime in your throat, a pimple or two, headache or felt bloated? That is usually because of a reaction to casein and/or lactose. Try to leave out all dairy products for six months, and slowly introduce them one by one. You will learn which one of the dairy groups you can handle. If you buy organic full-fat and grass-fed dairy products such as butter, yogurt and good cheese, you might be able to handle it better, once in a while.

I know we have been told for decades to drink milk 2-3 glasses a day to support our bones with calcium. Unfortunately that is not correct. In fact, countries with the highest consumption of milk, actually have the highest rate of osteoporosis and fractures, and countries with the lowest consumption of milk, have the lowest rate of osteoporosis and fractures.

The reason being is that we have to have a balance in our calcium/magnesium levels. If that balance is off you can develop osteoporosis. Adding too much calcium to our diet, means the body has to try and balance it out with magnesium. The biggest storage of magnesium is found in our bones and teeth. This means, to maintain the calcium/magnesium balance, you have to pull the magnesium from your bones and teeth. This will over time result in bone fractures, osteoporosis and tooth decay.

Milk has one purpose and one purpose only
- to make babies grow!

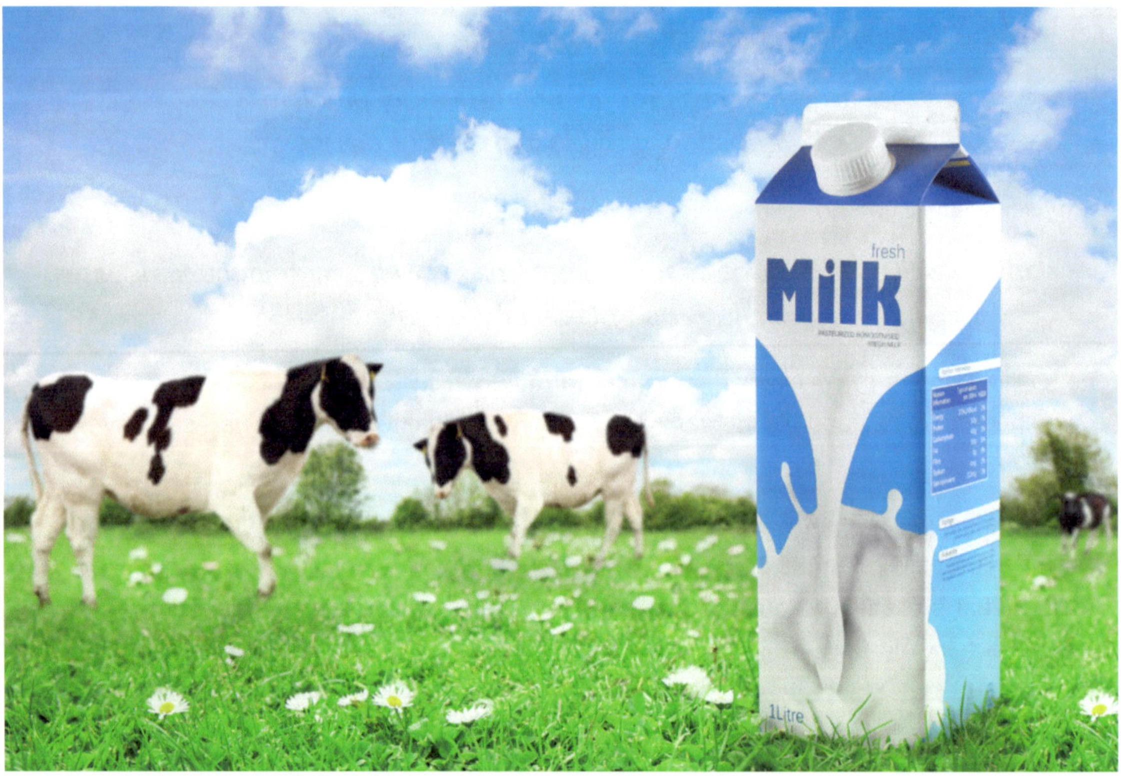

Goat cheese and sheep cheese on the other hand, have a lower casein content, and are therefore tolerated by most people. If you like yogurt, you can get dairy-free products like coconut milk, or almond milk yogurt which are both delicious.

Make sure to get the unsweetened original, to avoid any hidden sugars! Or even better, make your own. It's easy, delicious and a lot healthier than store bought.

Another reason to avoid dairy products is, they can have a cross reactivity with gluten, as it contains a similar protein as gluten. That's why I recommend no gluten or dairy for 6 months, before slowly introducing one thing at a time, to see how you react.
Use your Food, Body & Gratitude Journal to keep track of how and when you react to a food item. Get it at www.mygoodwitch.com/bookresources

A regular blood test will not show anything about sensitivity and intolerance for gluten and dairy, nor a cross reaction between the two. A delayed cross reaction can occur several hours after eating or drinking something.

Gluten

Just as it is the case with dairy, we are not designed to eat grain as we can get it today. We can eat nuts and most seeds, and they are a great substitute for grain. However, when we started using grain (seeds from different grasses) in our diet thousands of years ago, the plants were very different from the ones we get most grains from today. For example; the wheat we know today is often bred and genetically modified (GMO) over centuries, and provides absolutely no nutritional value for us. Gluten is a plant protein found in wheat, (all types including durum and spelt), ray and barley. This protein is what makes your bread airy. Unfortunately, gluten is a protein your body can't recognize and break down. Instead your body sees it as an external threat which activates your immune system to attack your own tissue, especially the intestine lining. This can go on for years, before you actually become aware something is wrong.

Remember, 60-70% of our immune system is found in our gut, especially the intestine lining as long as it is intact. When that lining breaks, inflammation and disease happens.

Leaky gut is one of them. This happens when the cells in the intestine lining are separated (they are usually locked like lego), and make room for microscopic particles of food to get into our bloodstream. This is one place they don't belong!

The latest research shows that anyone who consumes gluten, might have a leaky gut to some degree. Most of us have a Non Celiac Gluten Sensitivity, NCGS, which can cause the same diseases as if you have full blown celiac.

A review paper in The New England Journal of Medicine listed 55 diseases that can be caused by eating gluten. Here is just a few:

osteoporosis, irritable bowel syndrome, leaky gut, colitis,
anemia, cancer, fatigue, cold sores, rheumatoid arthritis, lupus, multiple sclerosis
and almost all other autoimmune diseases.

Gluten is also linked to many psychiatric and neurological diseases, including:

anxiety, depression, schizophrenia, dementia
migraines, epilepsy, neuropathy (nerve damage).

Most children with autism, ADD and ADHD do not tolerate dairy and gluten.

It might sound a little scary, but it is in fact reality. For example, when children with Autism or ADHD are fed gluten and/or dairy, they typically turn either hyper or apathetic.

Just think about it for a minute! How many kids wouldn't benefit from a clean diet with no gluten and dairy, instead of prescribing different medications! I am fully aware this is not a one type fits all solution. However, most will benefit positively from this approach.

As mentioned in the dairy section, you will not see if you benefit from a gluten and dairy free diet until you have completely cut it out for at least 6 months.

Unfortunately, that's how long it takes for your digestive system to rid itself of the autoimmune symptoms, inflammation and damage to the intestine lining caused by these foods.

In other words, if you eat as much as a cracker or some hidden gluten in restaurant food, you have to start all over.

And beware, gluten can be found in dressings, meats, breading, and even sushi! So in the beginning, you'll just have to read the labels, and when eating out, ask the waiter.

Unfortunately, that's also the case with celiac tests - which is only valid when your intestine walls are completely penetrated by gluten. Often, tests for celiac disease show false negatives because the patient is only experiencing partial gluten penetration.

Luckily you will soon learn to navigate the jungle of which products have gluten and hidden gluten, and come to enjoy all the amazing different gluten free options you have.

Fat & Fatty Acids

PLEASE forget everything you have heard for the past decades about eating low fat or no fat.

Fatty Acids play an important role in our health and are known as Essential Fatty Acids, meaning your body can not produce them on its own. You must get them through your diet.

You need a lot of fat to maintain or regain a healthy body and a balanced weight. It is therefore important to eat healthy fat, as well as the right ratio. A rule of thumb is, we need about 1/3 from each of the three main groups of fat, Mono-saturated-, poly-saturated-, and saturated fat.

Fatty Acids provide taste, nutrition, and energy to your body. Another good thing about fat is, it doesn't affect our blood sugar level the same way as carbs, it supports our cholesterol level, and it helps you lose weight. It also helps the absorption of fat soluble vitamins, A, D, E, and K, which all are critical for normal function, growth, and maintenance of tissues.

The following functions in your body all needs Fatty Acids for a flawless communication to maintain or regain optimal health:

cell membranes, brain health, immune system,
hormone system, heart health, nervous system, and joints.

Here is a couple examples:

Our brain is made of 60% fat - meaning, if you eat a diet with 0 fat, you starve your brain which will result in memory loss, concentration issues, and lower brain activity.

Your cell membranes (see illustration page 21) need fat in order for all the receptors and different signals to flow.

Another good thing about Fatty Acids is they don't affect your blood sugar level the same way as carbs, and they support your cholesterol level.

Processed Fatty Acids

It is important to remember refined and processed oils are NOT good for you. We now know this type of fat is causing:

chronic inflammation, diabetes, obesity, dementia, high cholesterol, as well as the risk of cancer.

This group includes butter spreads, margarine, crisco and all vegetable oil sprays, as well as the fats or oil in almost all processed foods.

Many restaurants use the cheaper types of oils, fats, and spreads for cooking. Unfortunately these don't tolerate high heat, if any heat at all, which will make them turn into trans-fats.

Trans-fat will cause oxidative stress, which over time will become diseases

Once you get used to the good and beneficial oils and fats, it is easy to taste the difference. All oil-fried foods are, in my opinion, toxic for you and should be avoided.

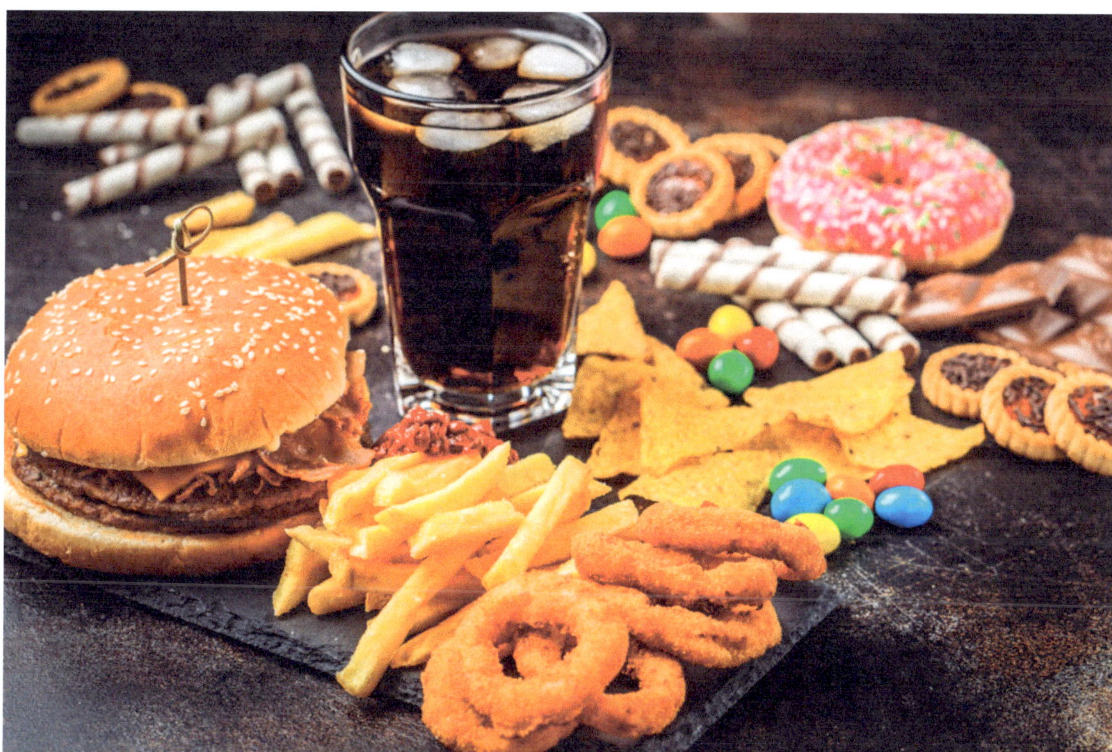

The Healthy Fatty Acids

As mentioned earlier you need all the omegas -3, -6 and -9 and about 1/3 from each group, monounsaturated-, polyunsaturated-, and saturated fat. Here is a short walk through the different types of fat.

Monounsaturated fat*

Omega 9 is a monounsaturated fat, and is actually produced in your body. You do also get it in your diet as oleic acid, as it is found in many different foods including nuts and seeds.

This group is known to help protect you against:

heart disease, lower your LDL cholesterol and blood pressure, as well as improve insulin sensitivity.

They are found in olive-, canola-, peanut-, sunflower- and safflower oils, as well as in avocados, peanut butter, and most nuts. It's also part of most animal fats such as fats from chicken, pork, and beef.

Polyunsaturated fat*

Omega 3 and Omega 6 fatty acids are polyunsaturated fats, and because they are liquid at room temperature, they are defined as oils.

This group is known to help:

reduce cholesterol levels and blood pressure, as well as help develop and maintain your body's cells. Last, they are essential for your brain function.

You find it in sunflower-, corn-, soybean- and cottonseed oils. It's also found in walnuts, pine nuts, flax-, sesame-, sunflower- and pumpkin seeds. You also get from sea food and grass fed animals.

* I would not recommend these two groups of oils and fat for cooking, as they don't tolerate high temperatures, except olive oil, which tolerates low heat. If they are used at high heat, they oxidize and turn into trans-fat, which is very harmful for you, as mentioned earlier.

Saturated fat

In this group you find the Omega 6 fatty acids. Despite what you have been told for the last decades, some saturated fats are actually GOOD for your health. Just like the mono- and polyunsaturated fat, the saturated fat also benefits your

brain health and cholesterol level. Furthermore it is supporting your immune system, nervous system, and bone health!

You find it in coconut oil, grass-fed butter, ghee, naturally raised animals, avocados, olives, nuts, and seeds. Coconut oil and avocado oil tolerate high heat and can be used for cooking.

Butter

Fortunately, you ***can*** have organic butter, and a lot of it, from grass fed cows.

Use it as gravy, make garlic or herb butter, and eat it for every meal if you want. Most people are better able to handle butter, versus other dairy products, because the proteins are easier to break down. However, stay away from all processed butter and margarine spreads. They will only provide more free radicals and oxidative stress in your body, which leads to disease.

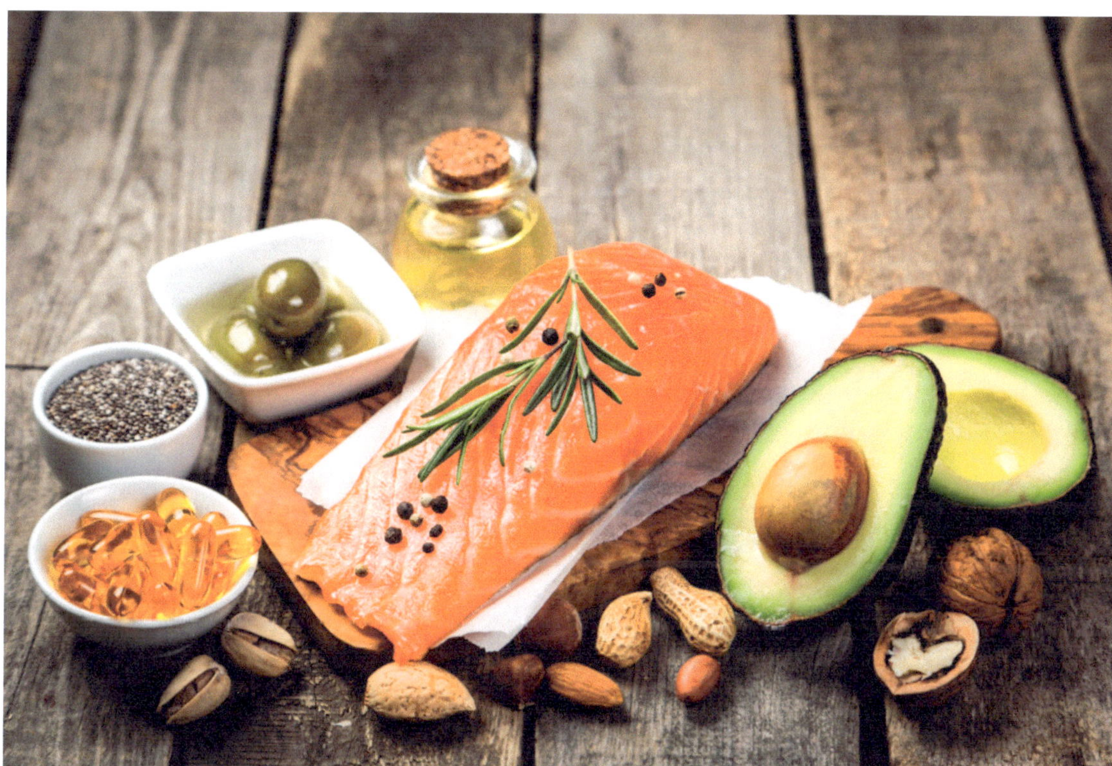

To Sum It Up

Everything we just went through in this chapter probably is a little overwhelming right now, and that is completely normal. That is why I have made it easy to navigate. When in doubt, go back and read it over and over. I promise, in a short time this will all become easy. You will quickly get to the point where you practice Mindful Eating, and only pick what nourishes you instead of breaking you down.

If you fall through the cracks once in a while, don't beat yourself up about it - just enjoy it, and get back at it the next day. The more you beat yourself up, the more you will deviate from your new lifestyle. Join our community on www.mygoodwitch.com/bookresources where you can ask questions and get support on your journey to a better quality of life.

Main things to remember about food

Ask yourself, is this good for me, or is it not good for me? And be honest with your answer.

Organic, grass-fed and wild caught meat, and locally grown, in season fruits and vegetables are all foods I highly recommend. Everything should be grown or raised without pesticides, herbicides, GMO, hormones, and medications.
When grocery shopping, shop the outer perimeter. This is where the food without labels is found.

Download the Mindful Eating Circle for easy access until it becomes second nature to you. You can find it at www.mygoodwitch.com/bookresources

"If the food hasn't been able to grow, walk, run, fly, or swim on its own - don't eat it"

Section Three
MINDFUL LIVING

You might not realize it, but stress and inflammation are major contributors to many health issues today.

These factors often go unnoticed even though they play a significant role in many of the lifestyle diseases we know today.

One powerful way to address these concerns is through mindful living. This approach encourages us to be more aware of our thoughts, feelings, and surroundings, and not just focusing on eating less and exercising more.

Chapter Ten

OUTDOORS

Fresh Air

Nothing beats the refreshing and calming power of fresh air. Try taking a walk in the morning or after dinner, and just breathe in the fresh air while listening to the birds. When you spend most of your time indoors in air-conditioned spaces, you're depriving your body of fresh air. This makes it harder for your body to stay energized and healthy.

Fresh air every day helps you clear your head, gives oxygen to your cells, and fills you with new energy. Go outside at least 30 minutes every day, regardless of the temperature!

Remember: it's not the weather, it's what you wear that matters!

Go for a walk, jog, run, bike ride, use your rollerblades, or whatever comes to mind. That also takes care of the exercise for the day :)

Some of the health benefits of fresh air are:

Good digestion

Fresh air increases the oxygen flow to your cells. This improves both the cell function, circulation, and helps you to digest your food more effectively.

If you are sitting a lot during your work day, more blood is directed to the brain. This may disrupt the digestion of food, and cause discomfort and indigestion. Try to go for a good walk outside after you eat.

Makes you happier

The fresh air you inhale, will help increase the oxygen in your blood. This means you get more oxygen to your brain, which then releases more serotonin.

Serotonin is your feel-good hormone, which lightens your mood, promotes happiness and well-being. Fresh air will also help increase your energy levels and clarity, as well as leave you refreshed and relaxed.

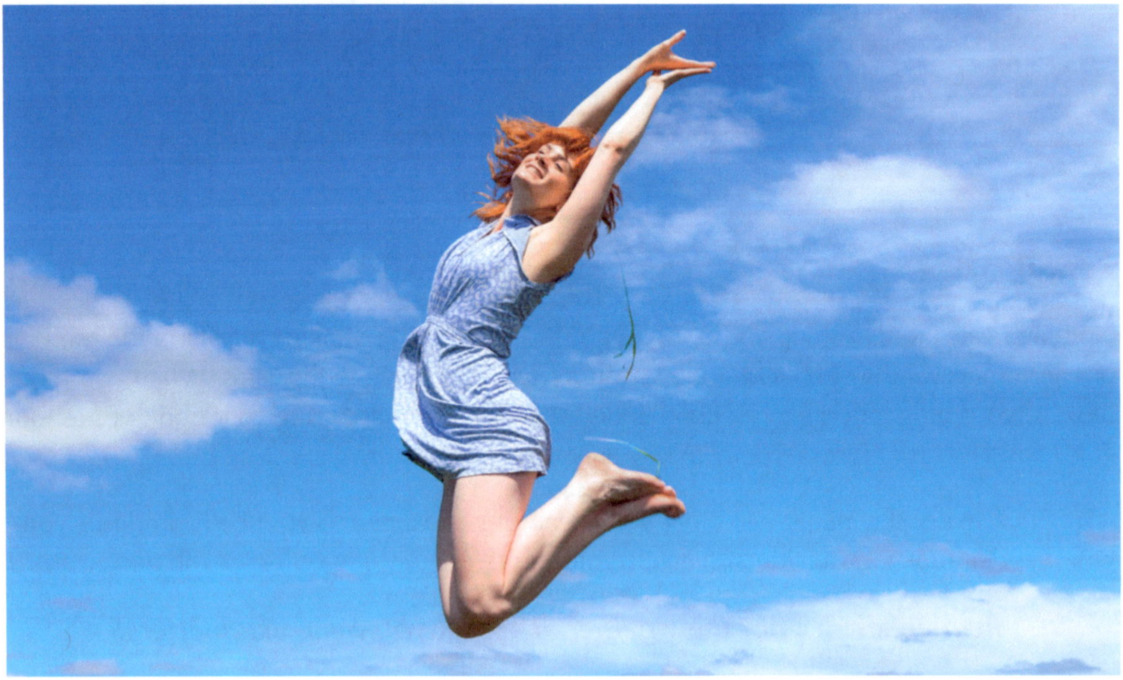

Strengthens your immune system

Every single cell in your body needs oxygen to do the metabolic process necessary to sustain life. Again, the more fresh air, the more oxygen to the body. Oxygen helps the white blood cells fight and eliminate harmful bacteria, viruses, parasites, and toxins.

Also the immune system is not able to maintain the inflammatory immune responses to keep the body protected without enough fresh oxygen.

Cleans your lungs

Indoor air, air conditioner air, or air in a highly-populated area is often a combination of nitrogen, carbon dioxide, and oxygen. This gives your lungs a hard time filtering out all the waste to provide you with sufficient amounts of oxygen.

Fresh air means more oxygen to your lungs, which helps your them by dilating the blood vessels, and causes the lungs to expand even more. The result is, when you exhale, you release airborne toxins from your body, and leave you with more energy.

Keeps your mind sharper

Fresh air helps you think better. More oxygen in your system means more oxygen to your brain. This improves your concentration and clarity. Your brain uses about 20% of your body's total oxygen!

One of my favorite benefits of going outside for a walk is how refreshed and full of energy and determination of getting stuff done I feel, once I'm back home. It is also a great way to clear your head, come up with ideas or solve a problem.

If the sun is shining while you're outside, you might even get some much needed Vitamin-D!

"Some old fashioned things like fresh air and sunshine are hard to beat"

~Laura Ingalls Wilder

Grounding

Grounding, or earthing, is something that was discovered by people like Dr. Clint Ober. He's a pioneer in this field and has done a lot of research on how it affects our well-being. Basically, grounding lets the earth's antioxidants enter our bodies and balance out harmful free radicals. This promotes a sense of balance and restores our natural energy. Dr. Ober's work has had a big impact and has started a global movement of people recognizing the benefits of grounding. This has also led to more research into how grounding can help our health.

Disconnection

There are several factors that contribute to our disconnection from grounding and hinder our ability to absorb the earth's energy. The main factor is the use of insulating shoes, which prevent the flow of electrons between our bodies and the earth. The use of rubber and plastic soles on shoes disrupt our connection to the earth's natural energy. Additionally, our modern lifestyle has confined us indoors, surrounded by synthetic materials that further insulate us from the earth's electrical charge.

Modern technology and the use of electronic devices also separate us from nature and limit our exposure to grounding. All of these factors combined contribute to the disconnection from grounding, depriving us of the potential health benefits it offers.

How To Do It

When we ground ourselves, the earth's negatively charged antioxidants enter our bodies and neutralize the positively charged free radicals within us. This process helps restore and promote our body's natural balance. In our modern lifestyle, we accumulate an abundance of free radicals and toxins, which can lead to imbalances and various health issues. These issues may manifest as feelings of being out of sorts, stressed, anxious, fatigued, depressed, or in pain.

If you are new to grounding, a simple way to start is to spend time outdoors barefoot or with direct skin contact to the earth's surface. Walking, standing, or sitting on grass, sand, or soil can help facilitate the flow of electrons from the earth into our bodies.

Start with 10 minutes and gradually increase the duration to 30 minutes per day.

Remember to choose conductive surfaces such as soil, grass, sand, or concrete, as these allow your body to draw energy from the earth. Surfaces like vinyl, wood, and asphalt are not conductive and will not provide the same benefits.

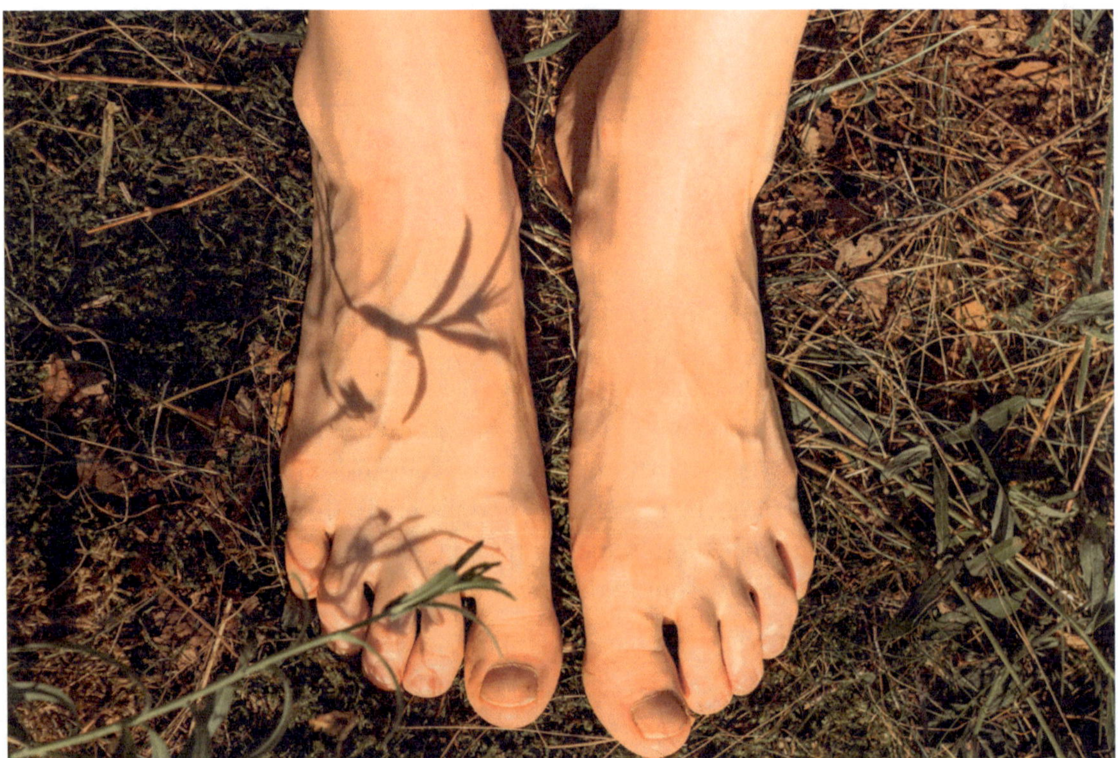

Also, prioritizing time in nature, away from cities and electromagnetically polluted areas; engaging in activities like gardening, hiking, or simply sitting under a tree, practicing yoga or meditation and regularly disconnecting from technology and spending time in nature, even just a few minutes a day will enhance the grounding experience.

Benefits Of Grounding

When you are grounded you will feel:

centered, less stressed, balanced, strong, and less tense. Additionally, grounding can provide pain relief, improve sleep quality, and enhance circulation.

In addition to these benefits, grounding has been associated with several other positive effects on health and well-being such as:

Reduced inflammation

Grounding has been found to have anti-inflammatory effects on the body. It can help reduce chronic inflammation, which is linked to various health conditions such as arthritis, cardiovascular disease, and autoimmune disorders.

Improved immune function

By reducing inflammation and promoting overall balance in the body, grounding can support a stronger immune system. This may help enhance the body's ability to fight off infections and diseases.

Enhanced mental clarity and focus

Grounding has been reported to improve cognitive function and mental clarity. It can help reduce brain fog, increase focus and concentration, and promote a greater sense of mental well-being.

Stress reduction

Grounding has a calming effect on the nervous system, helping to reduce stress and anxiety levels. It can promote relaxation, improve mood, and increase feelings of overall calmness.

Accelerated wound healing

Some studies suggest that grounding can aid in the healing process of wounds and injuries. It may help reduce pain, inflammation, and accelerate tissue repair.

Better sleep

Grounding has been associated with improved sleep quality. By promoting a state of relaxation and reducing stress, it can help individuals fall asleep faster, stay asleep longer, and wake up feeling more refreshed.

Balanced energy levels

Grounding is believed to help restore the body's natural energy balance. It can increase vitality, boost energy levels, and reduce feelings of fatigue and lethargy.

Tools used for grounding

Sometimes it is just not possible to go outside every day to do your grounding.

There are several tools available that can help you ground both outdoors and indoors. Here are some examples:

Grounding shoes

Grounding shoes, also known as earthing shoes, are designed to facilitate the practice of grounding even when walking or being outdoors. The benefits of grounding shoes is reconnecting with the earth's energy and to restore the natural energy balance in the body.

A side benefit of wearing grounding shoes is that you won't get zapped by touching things like car doors because your body stays uncharged. This is useful not just for cars but also in daily situations where static can build up, like using electronics, grabbing door handles, or touching metal surfaces. Grounding shoes keep you protected in different situations, making sure you stay safe from static shocks.

Grounding mats

These are specially designed mats that can be placed on the floor or on a desk. They are connected to the earth's grounding system through a cord, allowing you to experience the benefits of grounding while indoors. You can place your bare feet or hands on the mat to establish a connection with the earth's energy.

Grounding sheets

Similar to grounding mats, grounding sheets are made of conductive materials that are connected to the earth's grounding system. These sheets can be placed on your bed, allowing you to ground yourself while you sleep.

Grounding socks

These socks are made of conductive materials that allow the electrical charge from the earth to pass through to your feet. They are designed to be worn indoors and provide a grounding effect.

Grounding bands and wrist straps

These are wearable devices that you can wear around your wrist or ankle. They are equipped with conductive materials that establish a connection between your body and the earth's energy. These bands and straps are often used in workplaces where individuals are exposed to electronic devices for extended periods.

Exercise

It's incredibly important to incorporate exercise into your routines, preferably 3-5 times a week. But relax, it doesn't have to be 2+ hours each time! Exercise not only helps build muscles and strengthen the whole body. It also helps to let go of stored fat, support your digestive system, and move waste products out of the body.

The more you move during the day, the better your digestion will be to transport waste products out of the body. At the same time, sweat is a very good way of getting rid of waste products via your largest organ, the skin.

The lymphatic system also depends on exercise to function optimally. Lymph fluid is not pumped like our blood, but moves when the muscles squeeze the lymphatic system. When this happens, the lymph carries the white blood cells throughout the body, working to remove excess fat, bacteria, and other harmful materials.

By exercising regularly, your lymph stays active and flowing throughout your body, helping to carry out harmful waste products.

Exercise is also very important for your mood, as regular exercise helps to release endorphins, and these make you happier, more positive, and balanced in everyday life.

Even sleep is positively affected when you do regular exercise and your body can recover and recharge better for the next day.

All the above is why at least 30 minutes of daily exercise makes a huge difference.

Depending on your goals and body type, it's a good idea to incorporate these four different types of exercise into your program.

Cardio training

Running, biking, swimming, dancing - everything that's high-impact.
Improves your heart condition and provides a better blood flow throughout your body.

Strength training

Weight lifting, kettlebells, cross fit, or your own body weight.
Provides stronger bones and more muscles.

Balance or low impact

Yoga, Chai Chi, or just a stretching program. Provides a better reaction-time and coordination.

Breathing exercise

10 deep breaths 3 times daily. Relieves stress and provides oxygen to your cells.

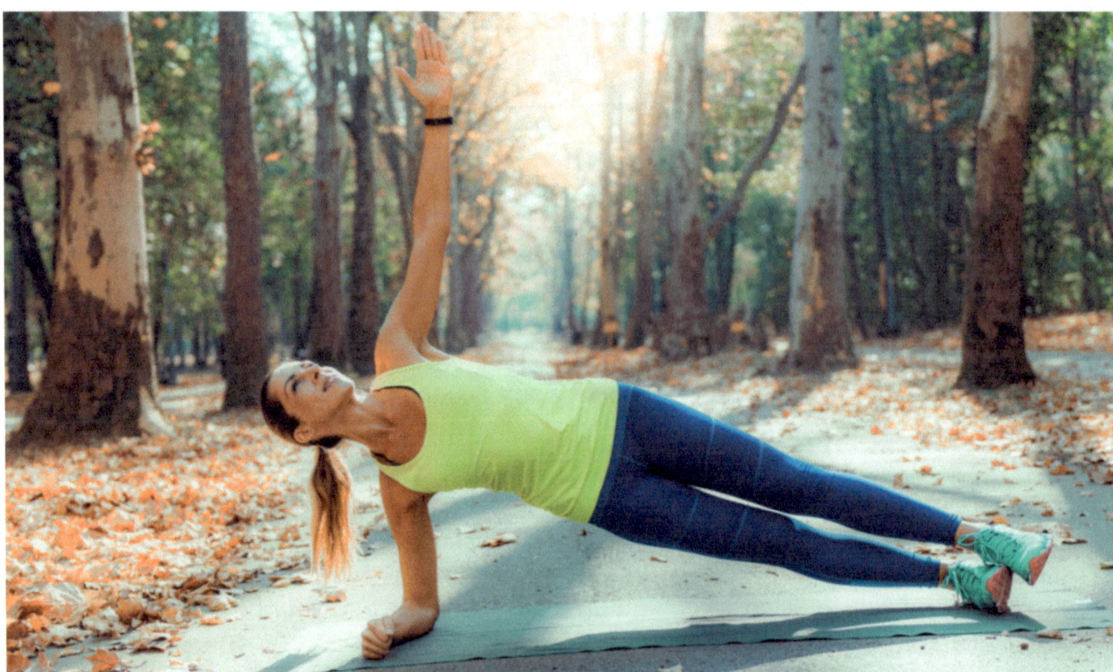

You can switch between the different types of exercise during the week. If you are having a hard time getting your exercise in, I highly recommend you join a fitness center. It's also a great idea to get a personal trainer in the beginning to keep you motivated and accountable.

I know you may think "I haven't got time for 3-5 hours of exercise a week" but let's be honest - how many hours do you watch television every day? If you give up just 30-60 minutes of television every day, you'd have plenty of time to exercise.

WARNING!
Exercise has been known to cause better
HEALTH AND HAPPINESS!

Chapter Eleven

SELF AWARENESS

Your health, beauty, and well-being is not just about what you eat, and how you exercise. Using the holistic approach, and working on you as a whole– body, mind, and spirit– you will turn old hidden patterns and suppressed memories into something useful and positive for you. Your positive attitude, self-love, and confidence will produce endorphins (your own happy hormones) which will inspire you to become even more aware of yourself, and committed to make positive changes.

You might not know this, but coherence and self awareness are both extremely important for you to succeed on your journey to optimal health. Changing your lifestyle is however everything but easy. And it is SO much more than eating the right food and doing your exercise.

To get a healthy foundation in place, I highly recommend implementing my "Seven Steps." This will teach fundamental inexpensive steps you can incorporate into your life on an everyday basis. Go back and read chapter 8 to get a feel for my "Seven Steps". You can also join my community to get the full version www.mygoodwitch.com/bookresources

This chapter will teach you how to work on your coherence and how to recognize the 4 levels of awareness.

It's an invaluable cognitive ability that distinguishes humans from other creatures. It empowers you to grow, build meaningful relationships, regulate your emotions, live authentically, make informed decisions, and contribute to a more harmonious society. This means you are able to recognize and understand your thoughts, emotions, motivations, and behaviors, and not only do you comprehend your own experiences but also consider how you impact others and the world around you.

Self-awareness is pivotal to human existence for several reasons. It is not merely an introspective exercise but a fundamental aspect of human existence, shaping your personal development and the world we create around us. Working on your self-awareness is a lifelong journey that gives you amazing rewards and ultimately enriches your own life as well as the lives of those around you. First and foremost, self-awareness is the cornerstone of personal growth and development. When you possess a deep understanding of yourself, you can identify your strengths and weaknesses, your preferences, and areas needing improvement.

This self-knowledge serves as a compass, guiding you toward making informed decisions, and setting meaningful goals. It empowers you to adapt, learn, and evolve, ultimately leading to personal growth and a sense of fulfillment.

Furthermore, self-awareness plays a pivotal role in having healthy relationships. Understanding your own emotions and motivations enables you to better comprehend the feelings and perspectives of others. This empathetic capacity enhances communication, empathy, and interpersonal skills, creating a foundation for strong and meaningful connections. In essence, self-awareness acts as a bridge, connecting yourself to others by promoting compassion and cooperation.

Self-awareness is also vital for emotional regulation. When you are aware of your emotions and the factors that trigger you, you are better equipped to manage your reactions and responses. This ability to self-regulate can prevent impulsive behavior and promote emotional stability, reducing the negative impacts of stress and anxiety on mental health.

In addition, self-awareness is closely tied to authenticity. When you are in touch with your true self, you can live in alignment with your values and beliefs. This authenticity fosters a sense of purpose and self-fulfillment, as you pursue paths that resonate with your core identity.

Moreover, self-awareness can have a positive impact on decision-making. It allows you to make choices that are congruent with your long-term goals and values, instead of giving in to what society expects or wants from you, or any short-term temptations. This capacity for informed decision-making can lead to a more fulfilling and purpose-driven life.

In the broader context of society, self-awareness can contribute to empathy and understanding among diverse groups. It promotes tolerance and open-mindedness as you become more aware of your own biases and prejudices. This, in turn, can lead to greater social connections.

The 4 Levels Of Awareness

The concept of self-awareness can be further understood through the lens of four distinct levels, each representing a different stage of personal development and consciousness

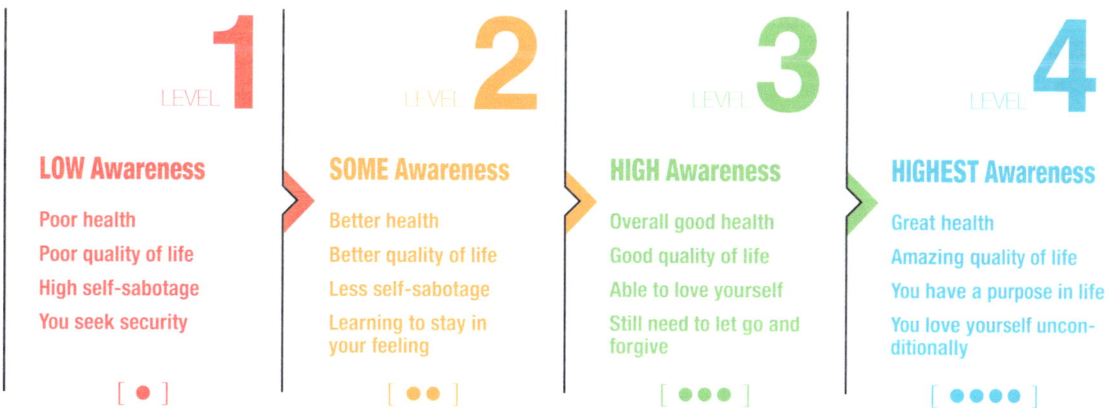
LEVEL 1
LOW Awareness
Poor health
Poor quality of life
High self-sabotage
You seek security
LEVEL 2
SOME Awareness
Better health
Better quality of life
Less self-sabotage
Learning to stay in your feeling
LEVEL 3
HIGH Awareness
Overall good health
Good quality of life
Able to love yourself
Still need to let go and forgive
LEVEL 4
HIGHEST Awareness
Great health
Amazing quality of life
You have a purpose in life
You love yourself unconditionally

Level 1: Low Awareness

At this initial stage, you may exhibit poor health, have a low quality of life, and often engage in self-sabotaging behaviors. Insecurity and self-doubt may dominate your thoughts and actions. You might find yourself trapped in a cycle of negative thought patterns and limited self-belief. Level 1 is marked by a lack of understanding of your own emotions, motivations, and your impact on life choices.

Level 2: Some Awareness

Moving beyond the limitations of Level 1, you begin to experience improvements in your health and overall quality of life. You become more attuned to your emotions and start to recognize the importance of staying present in your feelings rather than succumbing to self-sabotage. This level marks the beginning of a conscious effort to understand yourself better and make positive changes in life.

Level 3: High Awareness

At Level 3, you will achieve good health and an improved quality of life. You develop the capacity to love yourself, which is a significant milestone in self-awareness. However, even at this stage, there may be areas where you need to let go of past baggage and forgive yourself or others for past actions. When you have high awareness you have a deeper understanding of your motivations and emotions and are committed to personal growth and well-being.

Level 4: Highest Awareness

The highest level of self-awareness represents the pinnacle of personal development. At this stage you can enjoy great health and an amazing quality of life. You have not only learned to love yourself unconditionally but have also discovered a profound sense of purpose in life. This level brings you in a state of complete harmony and balance, where you have transcended many of the inner struggles you had at the lower awareness levels. You are not only in tune with yourself, you are also in harmony with the world around you and will be more conscious of the well being of others.

Knowing and using these 4 Levels Of Awareness is your road map for personal inner growth. It is a very transformative tool, allowing you to work with yourself from the state of insecurity and self-sabotage towards balance, purpose, and unconditional self-love. And remember, self-awareness is not the end destination - it's an ongoing journey of self-discovery and self-improvements which ultimately leads to a more harmonious and meaningful life.

Coherence

The more you work with yourself mentally, the more coherent (in balance) you'll become. If you are incoherent (out of balance) you will most likely experience sleeplessness, restlessness, and fatigue. You'll also become worrisome, foggy, apprehensive as well as have a negative mindset.

Being in this state will never get you the lifestyle you are working so hard to achieve. You might succeed for a period of time, but your old habits will slowly creep back into your life. When you are in coherence (in balance), you will experience mental clarity and peace, be energized, ready to conquer the world, and have a strong intuition.

How do you do it

Even if you've been self-sabotaging i.e beating yourself up about being overweight, always falling back into old habits, not liking what you see in the mirror, or thinking less of yourself, you will be alright. The mental work you will be doing will help you detox your brain, unblock your emotions, and regain vital energy.

Your brain is designed to ensure your survival. It needs to be involved and fed with positivity and confidence in order to avoid restoring old habits.

Though our instincts tell us that ***new things equal danger***, doing the inner work assures our instincts that our new lifestyle is ok.

You need to let go of what people think about you, and start believing that what you have to offer and what you stand for is authentic and true to you. The 4 Levels of Awareness will help you change your mindset and thoughts about yourself, including your surroundings, and help you to create a healthier, happier, and more beautiful version of you. Also you will become aware of things and relations that no longer fit you, and you will have no problem in letting them go. The more you work on this, the more natural it will become.

Gratitude

As mentioned earlier in my "Seven Steps", gratitude plays a huge role for your mental well-being. You may not always recognize things to be thankful for, but consider this: the fact that you woke up this morning, in itself, is a reason for gratitude. Just imagine the alternative – it wouldn't be very pleasant, right?

I encourage you to make a habit of jotting down at least five things you're grateful for each night before you go to bed. Use a paper journal, not your phone. Using a physical journal and writing things you're grateful for by hand, instead of on your phone, offers distinct benefits. It creates a tangible, mindful connection between your thoughts and paper.
The personal touch of handwritten entries also supports your memory and helps you reflect. It helps make your gratitude practice more emotional and unique to you.

Last but not least, the more you engage in this exercise, the more you'll discover just how much you actually have to be grateful for in your life. As gratitude journaling becomes a habit, you will not only have a more positive view on things, it will also boost your self awareness.

The Line Of Decision

This tool is simple yet powerful. It can help you become more self-aware, be more productive as well as help you have a positive attitude. Imagine this line as a clear boundary between two types of choices we can make in various situations.

Below The Line

This is where you consciously or subconsciously choose to act like a victim. You are making excuses, blaming others, procrastinating, and sabotaging yourself. When you do this, you give up control over your life, often without even realizing it. In other words, you fall below the line of decision.

Above The Line

This is where you choose to take ownership, accountability, and responsibility for your actions or lack thereof. You acknowledge that you have the power to influence your circumstances, even when life gets tough, and you recognize that your decisions and choices play a significant role in the outcomes.

Line Of Decision

you take ownership and responsibility, are accountable and acknowledge your circumstances good or bad.

Above The Line

↑

↓

Below The Line

You act like a victim, make excuses, blame others, procrastinating, and sabotaging yourself.

So, when you start working on your self-awareness, remember to be 100% true to yourself, and when in doubt, use the "line of decision." You will quickly learn to recognize when you are making excuses and when you are acknowledging your circumstance. It will help you be empowered to make conscious choices, being proactive when having challenges, and understanding that you have the ability to take control of your life. It's a reminder that you can navigate life's ups and downs with resilience and determination.

Ego says, "Once everything fall into place, I'll find peace"
Spirit says, "Find your peace, then everything will fall into place"

Your Inner Child

Working with your coherence and self awareness, you also work with your inner child.

Your inner child is a part of you that has been present ever since you were conceived, and has developed with you through the baby-, toddler- and childhood years. It can recall good experiences as well as childhood fears, neglect, losses, or traumas. In other words, your inner child is a part of your subconscious, and has been storing messages all along.

It holds emotions, memories, and beliefs from the past as well as dreams for the future.
When your inner child is running the show, you are what we call self sabotaging. This can be through fear, anxiety, perfectionism, or avoiding certain people, places, or situations. You (the inner child) will choose behaviors and thoughts based on unconscious beliefs or memories from the past.

Instead of self sabotaging, you will learn how to love yourself and your inner child for the wonderful and amazing person you are. Self awareness is about connecting to your inner child. It includes everything you learned and experienced as a child, before puberty. The inner child denotes a semi-independent entity subordinate to the waking conscious mind. Once you have restored that connection, you will be able to trust your gut feeling as well. You see, there is a huge connection between the brain, the heart, and the gut.

Oftentimes we neglect and sabotage ourselves for so long, that we are no longer connected to our gut feeling or instinct. Through reflection, and memory related exercises, you will learn how to reconnect with your inner child and how to stand strong in the person you are, knowing that you will make the right choices and decisions for you, at all times.

I am's

In order to reprogram your brain and belief system, another great tool is positive affirmations. Write down 15-20 positive and encouraging "I am" statements, and say them out loud in front of the mirror every morning.

"I am healthy, I am happy, I am fit, I am enough, I am successful"

When you say them out loud, you create a positive connection from mouth to ear, and your brain will start to overwrite old beliefs and increase your self esteem. Repeating these every day will create a positive way of thinking towards yourself, and you will start believing what your cells have known all along - ***you can do anything.***

Living The 4 Levels Of Awareness

Now it is time to go to work, and to be really honest and transparent with yourself. The "4 Levels of Awareness" is a tool you can use to recognize where your self awareness is at, and how you can improve it to the highest level. You will be surprised to see how spot-on these levels of awareness are. Please remember the line of decision. Don't get trapped in the victim of circumstance. Work your way through it by addressing the real source of your problem or mental blockage.

To support you through this self-awareness journey, I've created a Food, Body & Gratitude journal which is a simple tool for you to document your daily observations across the 4 levels and your lifestyle change in general. Find it on www.mygoodwitch.com/bookresources

The more you track your daily activities and emotions, the easier it becomes to pinpoint what's happening in your body and mind. Through this process, you'll feel discomfort, recognize different triggers, and negative habits. I hope you find this tool helpful and get inspired to initiate positive changes.

***"Self-awareness is the key to personal growth.
By understanding who you are, your strengths and weaknesses,
you lay the foundation for true wisdom and a fulfilling life."***

~Birgitte Haaning Christensen

LEVEL 1

LOW Awareness

Poor health

Poor quality of life

High self-sabotage

You seek security

[•]

Level 1 - Low Awareness

Living by your EGO rather than your heart can lead to a range of challenges. It often manifests as poor health, a diminished quality of life, low self-esteem, and a tendency towards frequent self-sabotage. In such a state, the quest for security becomes a constant, desperate search from external sources.

This way of living keeps you trapped in a cycle where fundamental human needs, such as eating when hungry, sleeping when tired, or responding promptly to bodily cues, are neglected. Breaking free from this pattern requires a fresh start, rebuilding a foundation of comfort, and rediscovering self-love and trust. It's an essential journey to break free from the limitations imposed by an ego-driven existence and embrace a more fulfilling and authentic life guided by the heart.

Physical

Physically, the impact of living with an ego-driven mindset is evident. Blocked energy becomes a tangible issue, manifested through challenges such as being overweight, experiencing fatigue, constipation, various pains, and heightened stress levels. Skin concerns, whether oily or dry, recurrent illnesses, cellulitis, and edema further underscore the toll this lifestyle takes on your well-being.

In coping with these challenges, turning to comfort foods often becomes a default response, with a reliance on sugar, carbs, and other nutritionally lacking options. Additionally, your approach to exercise tends to be intense, driven by a strong desire to meet ambitious goals.

The self-sabotaging whispers of your ego contribute to this cycle, echoing sentiments like "I'm fat," "I'm not worthy," "I'm ugly," and "I don't have willpower." Breaking free from these patterns involves addressing not just the physical symptoms but also nurturing a mindset that fosters self-love, acceptance, and a more balanced approach to well-being.

Psychological

On the psychological front, your existence is stuck in a fight-or-flight survival mode. This state of being often obscures your awareness of self-sabotaging tendencies, leaving you uncertain about what is truly beneficial or detrimental for your well-being. The signals from your body go unnoticed, and you find yourself making excuses to rationalize unhealthy habits. Whether it's considering things too challenging, costly, time-consuming, or expressing preferences about breakfast choices and pill swallowing, these justifications become shields against acknowledging and addressing deeper issues.

Assigning blame to your surroundings for perceived shortcomings becomes a common reflex, fostering a sense of self-pity and a belief that you are missing out on life. In this state, you may feel disconnected from others, experiencing loneliness, a pervasive sense of being lost, and confusion.

During periods of low awareness, you tend to develop a reliance on external systems, books, and guidance from others instead of trusting your own instincts. Breaking free from this pattern involves not only recognizing these behaviors but also cultivating a deeper connection with yourself and building the confidence to trust your inner wisdom.

Thoughts and facts

When it comes to your thoughts and facts, you tend to be more talkative, often neglecting the art of listening.

Your conversations are often filled with negativity, centered around complaints about your circumstances, your spouse, kids, friends, and work. Rather than seeking solutions, you are looking for faults. Engaging in conflicts and holding opinions about everything and everyone is a common theme. The tendency to blame and accuse others for your emotional state or life situation is a characteristic of this phase.

Your ego plays a role in coming up with excuses, serving as justifications for the lack of progress. It feels like you're stuck in a cycle of conflict and drama, with an imaginary sense of lacking support from others.

In this state, there may be a lack of awareness that your surroundings act as a mirror reflecting the resistance and lack of self-support within you. Recognizing that you're trapped in an illusion about the past and the future is a crucial step toward breaking free from this pattern.

Past illusions

"I used to weigh 20 lbs less," "You should have known me when I was super fit."

You are also most likely saving clothing that's either too big or too small.

Future illusions

"When the kids are grown up… 'I'll have made more money; I will retire; I'll lose weight; You'll see me live out my dreams, train more, make better food choices!"

You have to remember, these are all illusions!

If you want to see how your future looks if you don't make changes now, then you just take a look at your past, because that is exactly how your future will look!

Scary right? If you want change, be the change. Take responsibility for your life, and trust yourself. It's time to move on. Being at this level is a cry for help from your body and your inner child. Picture yourself as a little newborn baby, who is cold, hungry, and crying. What does this baby need? The most basic fundamentals such as warmth, love, food, sleep, etc. You have to learn to give that to yourself again.

Go to the bathroom as soon as you feel you have to go. Eat when you are hungry. Rest when you are tired. Drink when you are thirsty. Love and appreciate yourself just the way you are.

It's all about becoming whole again, and only you can fill the gap by pouring love and attention into your inner child.

LEVEL 2

SOME Awareness

Better health

Better quality of life

Less self-sabotage

Learning to stay in your feeling

[●●]

Level 2 - Some Awareness

Your well-being and quality of life are getting better. You're starting to notice when you sabotage yourself and are figuring out how to stay in touch with your feelings. Now, you realize that there's a part of you that wants to change and another part that doesn't. But don't worry, It's simply a battle between your two EGOS!

Doing the self-sabotage exercise at this stage will help you move forward. Write down the negative emotions in your Food, Body & Gratitude Journal immediately whey they occur, and you will soon begin to identify when you shift between positive and negative emotions.

Gradually, you'll get better at expressing exactly how you feel and saying no when you mean it. You're on your way to healing!

Physical

Physically, a new awareness is growing within you. Your body is communicating a new language– one that you're just beginning to understand. As you slowly change your diet, lifestyle, and habits, you will experience a positive change and you find yourself feeling better. The positive changes take root, and old aches and pains gradually fade away.

This phase can be both exciting and frightening at the same time. The temptation to stay in Level 1 is strong, as there's a tendency to self-sabotage in order to avoid the perceived pain and effort tied to making lifestyle changes.

However, acknowledging this pattern is a crucial step in overcoming it and embracing the positive transformations underway.

Psychological

Your emotional healing is underway, and you're starting to understand the price both you and your family paid during the time you were stuck at Level 1. At that level, you shut down not only the painful emotions but also the beautiful and loving ones. This explains the rollercoaster of feeling awesome one day and everything sucking the next!

Now, you're conscious of the lack of awareness you had in level 1 and how it was draining your life and passion. This realization can be quite painful. Recognizing these shifts and understanding that your EGO doesn't always work in your favor is all part of the healing process, and you're well on your way to the next level.

Thoughts and facts

Soon, you'll come to the realization that everything your surroundings reflect is a mirror of your internal state. It's time to step up and take responsibility!

When faced with resistance, ask yourself, "Who is questioning you, criticizing you, misunderstanding you, and taking care of you?"

Dig deep and be brutally honest with yourself. From there, purposefully consider how you can enhance your self-care, amplify self-love, and achieve balance. Embrace the lessons mirrored by your surroundings and make intentional strides toward personal growth.

Traps

At Level 2, it's common to experience past issues and emotions from your childhood that you thought were already resolved. This isn't a setback; rather, it's a clear indication that you're progressing toward the next level.

You'll likely face temptations from various directions - new projects, the desire for a new home, a dog, or a vacation. Old relationships might resurface, as well as previous patterns or conflicts. Consider all of these occurrences as tests to determine whether you're prepared to move forward or if a part of you is still stuck to Level 1. Stay strong and don't let these challenges get to you.

Why are you at this level and what does it mean?

This level marks a crucial step in your journey toward optimal health. Having laid the groundwork and moved from Level 1, it's now time to rebuild!

You're in the process of rediscovering and truly experiencing life, and using your Food, Body & Gratitude journal you are now getting to know and FEEL yourself again - embracing both the joy and the pain. Handling your emotions can be a mentally exhausting and time consuming process. Resist the urge to stop midway due to fears of encountering love, vulnerability, excitement, or pain. Doing so only creates a toxic environment and leads to blocked energy. Keep moving forward in your healing journey.

How do you move on

By staying in your feelings, experiencing them fully, and addressing them authentically and vulnerably, you pave the way for progress. A crucial shift in mindset is alpha and omega!

Here's an example:

When your EGO tries to dominate with negative thoughts, counteract it by jotting down 10 positive things you're grateful for. As you cultivate this new positive mindset, you'll be prepared to advance to Level 3, where you'll master the art of letting go of things that are holding you back!

LEVEL 3

HIGH Awareness

Overall good health

Good quality of life

Able to love yourself

Still need to let go and forgive

[●●●]

Level 3 - High Awareness

Your well-being and quality of life have reached a positive state. Now, you can genuinely love yourself, and your ability to stay in touch with your feelings has grown.

At this level, the lesson is about releasing old habits and shedding negative emotions to make room for the new and positive. Use your *Food, Body & Gratitude Journal* to write down those negative emotions.

Stepping out of your comfort zone involves distancing yourself from addictions such as shopping, sugar, alcohol, cigarettes, and excessive attention-seeking.

To fully embrace life and share its joys with those around you, forgiveness and letting go of the last remnants of your past are essential. Once accomplished, you're ready to ascend to the highest level of awareness.

Physical

At this level, the focus is on detoxifying, releasing, and forgiving. While undergoing these processes, you might notice a temporary change in body odor that may not be pleasant. Check out my detox tools in chapter twelve.

Physical transformations will manifest as you shed fat and build muscle. You might have a brief feeling of weight gain, but it's part of the process. Stay committed to your newfound routines from my "Seven Steps".

During this period, it's crucial to flood your body with fresh vegetables. I recommend incorporating some form of vegetables into all three meals - whether raw, stir-fried, boiled, or grilled.

Psychological

Trust is key! This level of awareness requires all of your courage. You'll experience your power and fill yourself with energy and joy from the inside out.

If you've ever felt like pouring from an empty cup in the past, now is the moment to fill it up and take action. Only **YOU** can do that!

If you still feel the need for control and acceptance from others, it's time to **LET IT GO** and experience the bubbling excitement within. Release the habits of judging, frustration, addiction, and pettiness.

This journey is about embracing understanding, compassion, and a sense of belonging, so let go of the fight for good.

Thoughts and facts

Letting go of old patterns and emotions can be challenging since they've been a part of your perception of yourself. It's like letting go of who you believed you were!

The feeling you'll experience when you truly feel, love, and believe in yourself will be both euphoric and intimidating. Stay committed to your efforts, and you'll find yourself at level 4 sooner than you think!

Wake up call

If you still feel some bitterness, addiction, jealousy, or conflict, it's essential to revisit Level 1 or 2 to address unresolved conflicts. The more you write down in your journal and honestly share every aspect of yourself - your vulnerabilities, deepest secrets, and sides you'd rather keep hidden - the closer you are to Level 4. Doing so, you'll realize a gradual reduction in conflicts, drama, and fights, replaced by a genuine interest and curiosity in yourself, friends, and family. The people around you will undergo changes, offering unexpected support and attention as they recognize and appreciate your transformations.

By embracing authenticity, balance, and self-love, you not only heal yourself but also positively influence those around you. This approach opens new doors and creates opportunities, shifting the focus from obstacles and negativity.

Traps

Don’t be tempted to think less about your accomplishments. True appreciation and thankfulness for your journey will create healthy cells! If you don’t acknowledge your amazing changes, you will end up right back at Level 1. Love yourself and be proud of yourself. The biggest fear at this level is still not knowing who you will become when you have completed your change.

How do you move on

By letting go, decluttering, and throwing out everything that doesn't serve you anymore, both physically and mentally, you will be able to truly trust yourself. Just remember, everything you hold on to is holding you back.

Recognize that your comfort zone is a temporary security, and that true growth only comes from stepping outside of it. When you have let go of everything that is no longer serving you, you are ready to move on to the final level.

LEVEL 4

HIGHEST Awareness

Great health

Amazing quality of life

You have a purpose in life

You love yourself unconditionally

[●●●●]

Level 4 - Highest Awareness

Your well-being and life quality are extraordinary. You have strength, vitality, and are in perfect balance.

By stepping out of your comfort zone, you've taken responsibility by prioritizing yourself and your needs, having unconditional self-love, and attentively listening to your gut feelings.

Knowing your life's purpose, you now stand firm in your emotions. It becomes clear that those around you are inspired to replicate your actions and embody who you are.

Physical

Your digestive system, endocrine system, and nervous system operate with excellence, you've acquired the knowledge to effectively manage physical discomfort, whether it be through dietary adjustments or seeking therapeutic relief such as massage therapy. Due to your consistency in journaling, you now have heightened awareness and a proactive approach to maintaining well-being.

Psychological

At this level, everything effortlessly aligns, and you've learned to enjoy and appreciate all the goodness that comes your way. The law of attraction is now an integrated part of your daily life. You exist in coherence, maintaining a positive and open mindset while being surrounded by inspiring and like minded people.

With a solid foundation, any fall backs to old patterns are corrected immediately, and stability is regained. Your strong foundation allows you to design the life you desire through your passion. The positive impact of your transformative changes is palpable.

Thoughts and facts

Now you have all the tools you need to keep yourself at this level. You feel balanced and successful, and the positive changes from your journey show in every part of your life.

Wake up call

If you notice yourself slipping from your new level of balance and awareness, you are now able to catch it immediately. It usually starts with doubting your own abilities and/or stressing about your finances. To fix this, go back to Levels 1, 2, and 3 to figure out what issues you need to deal with. It might be basic things like getting enough sleep, eating well, staying hydrated, or attending to bathroom needs. Listen to what your body is telling you, and you'll quickly find yourself back at Level 4.

Relationships with yourself

The transformations happening around you are a result of the shifts in your perspective.

Go with the flow and enjoy the new you - the balance you've found and the better understanding of what's good for you. It's clear that being at this higher awareness level takes effort and might feel a bit lonely at times. You're always taking responsibility, and you know that avoiding challenges by getting lost in work, family, relationships, or excuses isn't an option anymore.

Traps

Don't take these positive changes in your lifestyle, health, and well-being for granted. It's so easy to forget how drained and closed up you were back in Level 1.

If you hear those little voices suggesting it's okay to take a few steps back, resist! Going back might lead you into self-sabotage. Keep working on the reflections - what you project back to yourself - and continue appreciating and loving yourself.

To stay at this highest level of awareness, keep doing what you're doing now. Being in balance and maintaining your foundation is your new normal. When challenges arise, you know exactly how to react and deal with them. You listen to your inner voice and love yourself unconditionally.

You've reached the highest level of awareness, and now, you're the best possible version of yourself, living a fulfilled life.

Knowing your life's purpose, you now stand firm in your emotions. It becomes clear that those around you are inspired to replicate your actions and embody who you are.

Chapter Twelve

DETOX

Taking care of our health has never been more crucial, especially in today's fast-paced and often toxin-filled world. Detoxification, also known as Detox, is a process that helps rid our bodies of harmful substances. It plays a vital role in promoting overall well-being. In this chapter, we'll explore the importance of detox and share practical tools that you can effortlessly implement at home, without spending a fortune.

Our bodies are constantly exposed to a variety of toxins from numerous sources, including non-organic foods, chlorine, and fluorides in drinking water, mercury from dental fillings and thermometers, lead from pipes and smoldering materials, hormone disruptors such as BPA and phthalates aluminum from tinfoil and environmental toxins like EMF and Wi-Fi radiation.

These harmful substances infiltrate our tissues and cells, and long time exposure can have huge negative effects on our metabolism, behavior, immune system, and overall brain health.

The consequences of toxicity can manifest in many different symptoms, including fatigue, joint pain, headaches, digestive imbalances, sleep disorders, and mental health issues.

Furthermore, it can contribute to the development of serious illnesses like Alzheimer's, multiple sclerosis, and Parkinson's disease. To optimize your well-being and rid your body of these harmful toxins, it is very important to take action and start detoxing.

The Simple Detox Tools offer a multitude of benefits:

immune support, toxin eliminations, weight loss support, increased energy, improved skin, chronic disease prevention, and improved mental and emotional clarity.

Incorporating the Simple Detox Tools is a proactive step towards achieving and maintaining better health, allowing you to enjoy a more vibrant and fulfilling life, while also effectively addressing the modern challenges posed by hormone disruptors, environmental toxins, and electromagnetic radiation from Wi-Fi.

My Simple Detox Tools

The Simple Detox Tools I have used and shared over the years include a variety of supplements and oils, which can help absorb and eliminate toxins from your body. Additionally, easy-to-do detox methods you can try at home include oil-pulling, where you swish coconut oil in your mouth to remove oral toxins, detox drinks made from natural ingredients, foot baths to pull out toxins, and dry brushing your skin to stimulate lymphatic drainage and exfoliate dead skin cells. These accessible and effective tools make detox a practical and achievable part of your daily routine.

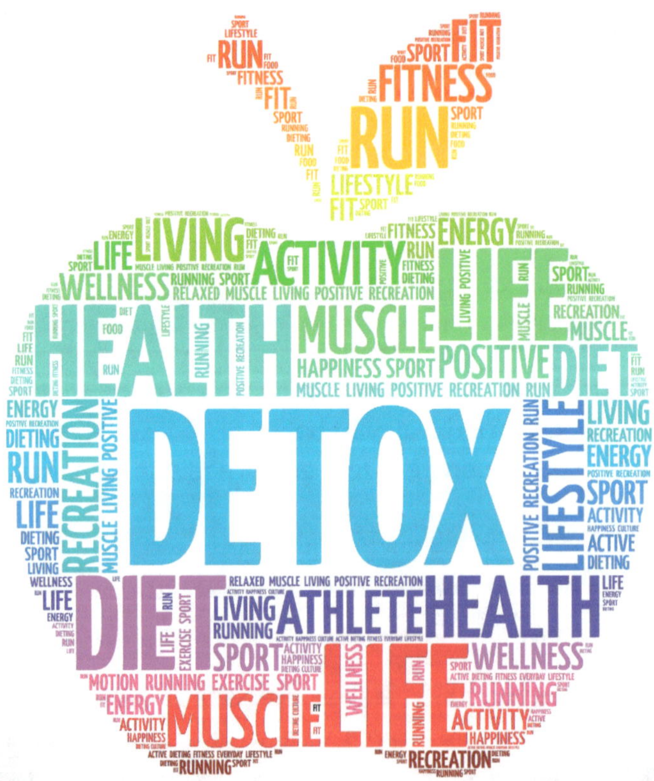

Oil Pulling

Oil pulling is deeply rooted in the ancient tradition of Ayurvedic medicine, which dates back thousands of years in India.

In Ayurveda, the practice of oil pulling, known as "kavala" or "gundusha," is considered a powerful method for promoting oral and systemic health. The therapeutic benefits of oil pulling, describing it as a means to purify the entire body by drawing out toxins and impurities.

The practice is believed to balance the fundamental energies and enhance overall well-being. Ayurvedic practitioners have long recognized the connection between oral health and systemic health, making oil pulling a cornerstone of holistic wellness within this ancient healing system.

Today, oil pulling continues to gain popularity for its potential to support oral hygiene and overall detox.

When you start oil pulling it is important to use organic unrefined coconut oil, because it provides a more natural, pure, and high-quality product that is free from synthetic chemicals and additives. It not only offers potential health benefits but also aligns with environmentally sustainable practices and avoids the use of chemicals like hexane.

Organic unrefined coconut oil is made from fresh coconut meat that is cold-pressed or expeller-pressed, and it doesn't undergo the refining and chemical processing that refined coconut oil does. This results in a purer, more natural product with higher quality and with its natural nutrients, flavor, and aroma. It also has a richer, more authentic coconut flavor and aroma compared to refined coconut oil, which may have a neutral taste or a more processed smell and taste.

When choosing organic coconut oil, you also support environmentally friendly and sustainable farming practices. Organic farming methods prioritize soil health, biodiversity, and reduced chemical usage, contributing to a healthier planet.

Last but not least, organic coconut oil is non-GMO, meaning it is not genetically modified. This ensures that the coconuts used to make the oil are grown naturally, without genetic engineering.

How does it work

Oil pulling activates saliva enzymes that absorb and neutralize various toxins, including chemical and environmental pollutants, as well as bacterial byproducts. As these harmful substances are expelled through the tongue during the oil pulling practice, they are no longer a threat to your health. This holistic approach to well-being extends beyond just oral health; it can potentially offer relief from common ailments by reducing the overall toxic burden on the body.

By lessening the load of these toxins, oil pulling assists in achieving a state of better balance and health. Following are some of the benefits you can experience by adding oil pulling to your daily routine.

Excretion of Toxic Heavy Metals

Oil pulling helps the excretion of toxic heavy metals through saliva. This process activates salivary enzymes that absorb a range of toxins, including chemical, bacterial, and environmental toxins, purging them from the bloodstream and expelling them through the tongue.

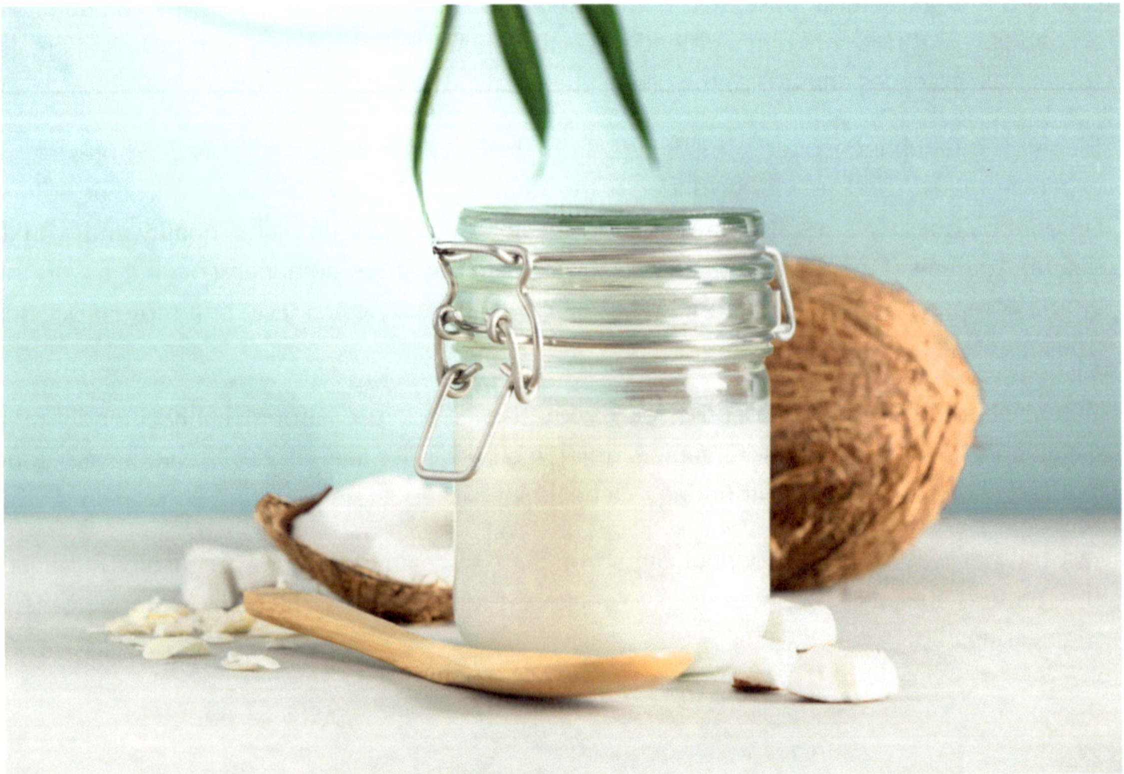

Oral Health Benefits

Oil pulling offers several benefits for your oral health. It helps whiten your teeth, promotes fresh breath, and supports gum health. By swishing the oil thoroughly in your mouth, you can also target specific areas, such as between teeth and around the gums, to enhance your dental well-being.

Additional benefits of Oil pulling is reduced oral bacteria load which have a positive influence on the immune system and your gut health. This means you will most likely see reliefs in headaches, allergies and skin conditions like acne, eczema, psoriasis, dry skin and dull complexion.

As the oil is swished around the mouth, it acts as a natural detoxifier, binding to toxins, bacteria, and impurities that can accumulate in the oral cavity.

Step By Step

To incorporate oil pulling into your routine, start by following these few steps:

- Start by taking a tablespoon of coconut oil into your mouth
- Begin swishing the oil around inside your mouth. You can start with just 5 minutes, especially if you're new to oil pulling. Gradually, work your way up to 15-20 minutes as you become more comfortable with the process.
- As you swish the oil, make sure to cover your entire mouth. This means moving it around the front and back of your mouth, over your tongue, and toward the back of your throat.
- During the swishing process, try to keep the oil moving consistently and avoid swallowing it. Swallowing the oil prematurely may defeat the purpose of the practice.
- After the recommended swishing time, spit the oil out into a trash can. Avoid spitting it into the sink, as coconut oil solidifies when coming in contact with cold water and can therefore clog drains over time.
- Finally, rinse your mouth thoroughly with warm water to remove any remaining oil residue.

With its roots in ancient traditions and a constantly growing amount of scientific evidence, oil pulling continues to gain popularity as an inexpensive tool for detox and wellness practice you can do from the comfort of your home.

Detox Drinks

Starting your day with a glass of water infused with either lemon juice or apple cider vinegar has gained popularity in recent years for good reason. This morning ritual offers a refreshing and detoxifying kickstart to your system. But what is the difference between the two?

Lemon juice is derived from fresh lemons and primarily consists of water and citric acid. It is prized for its high vitamin C content, hydration, alkalizing effect, and antioxidant properties, and is excellent for promoting immune health, aiding digestion, and gentle detox.

Apple cider vinegar *(ACV)* is made from fermented apple juice and contains acetic acid, which gives it its distinctive sour taste. For centuries ACV has been used as a health-promoting agent, because of its high levels of vitamin B and C, as well as polyphenols, antioxidants and acetic acid, which increase the absorption of minerals from the foods we eat, and slow down the conversion of carbohydrates into sugar. On the other hand, apple cider vinegar is known for its potential to improve digestion, stabilize blood sugar, assist in weight management, and support heart health.

Here's why they are an important tool in your quest to eliminate toxins from your body.

Hydration

First and foremost, hydrating your body after a night's sleep is crucial. Water is essential for overall health and is involved in countless bodily processes, including digestion and the elimination of waste. Adding lemon or ACV to your water makes it more appealing, encouraging you to drink more and stay hydrated.

Digestive Aid

Both lemon juice and apple cider vinegar are known for their digestive benefits. Lemon contains citric acid, which can stimulate the production of digestive enzymes, helping your stomach break down food more effectively. ACV, on the other hand, contains acetic acid, which may improve digestion and nutrient absorption.

Alkalizing Effect

Although lemon juice is acidic, it has an alkalizing effect on the body when metabolized. An alkaline environment is believed to be less conducive to the growth of harmful microorganisms and may help maintain a balanced pH level in the body.

Liver Support

Lemon juice and apple cider vinegar are thought to support the liver, the body's primary detoxification organ. These substances may enhance the liver's ability to flush out toxins, promoting optimal liver function.

Antioxidant

Lemons are rich in vitamin C, a powerful antioxidant that can help combat free radicals in the body. This antioxidant action may contribute to reducing oxidative stress and inflammation, supporting overall health.

Detoxification

Lemon juice and ACV can act as natural diuretics, promoting urine production and flushing out waste and toxins from the body. This gentle detox process helps alleviate bloating and leaves you with a feeling of lightness.

To incorporate this morning ritual into your routine, simply squeeze the juice of half a lemon or add a tablespoon of ACV to a glass of warm water. Drink it on an empty stomach before consuming any food or beverages. You will experience improved digestion, increased energy, and a greater sense of well-being as your body benefits from the detox effects of this simple yet powerful practice.

Cranberry Juice

Mixing raw cranberry juice with lemon juice and ACV, is a powerful natural detox drink that benefits multiple organs and systems in your body. Cranberries are packed with nutrients and antioxidants, such as vitamin C and flavonoids, known for their ability to support the removal of fats from the lymphatic system. This system plays a crucial role in absorbing fats from your digestive system and transporting them to the bloodstream.

Keeping your lymphatic system clean and functional is vital for overall health, as it not only helps with fat transport but also in removing harmful toxins from the kidneys, liver, and bowels. This very simple and powerful combination of ingredients supports your body's natural detox processes and helps you towards optimal health and well-being.

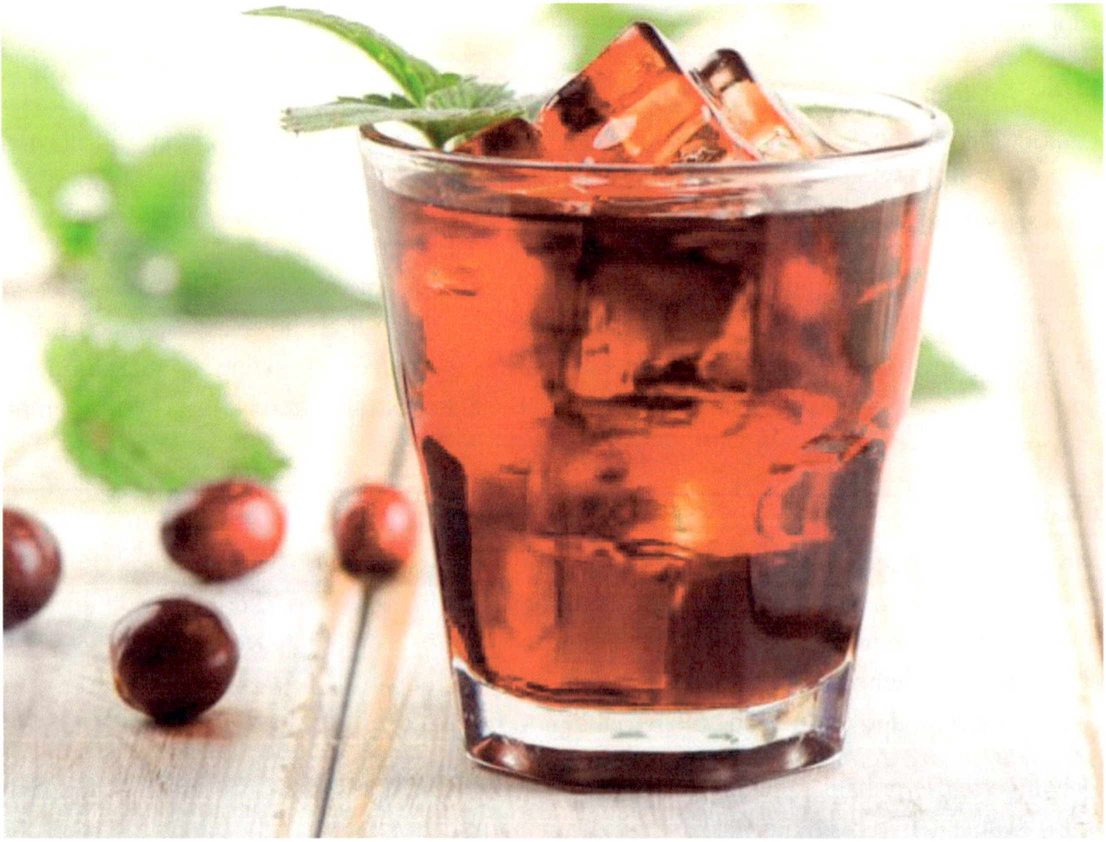

How To Do It

Throughout the year, rotate Lemon juice and water, ACV and water, and the Cranberry mix 2-4 weeks. It is a smart approach to maintain the effectiveness of your detox routine.

Your body has a remarkable ability to adapt to consistent patterns, including dietary habits. By rotating the detox drinks regularly, you prevent your body from getting accustomed to one specific blend, which might diminish its impact over time.

Each drink targets different toxins and aspects of detox, ensuring a more comprehensive cleansing of your organs and systems. This rotation not only keeps your detox regimen fresh and interesting but also maximizes the benefits, helping you achieve and maintain optimal health and vitality.

When you are done with the oil pulling, and before breakfast drink one of these detox drinks.

Mix one of the following:

Lemon & Water Drink

2 tbsp of organic Lemon Juice
8 oz of filtered water.

Apple Cider Vinegar & Water Drink

2 tbsp of ACV
8 oz of filtered water

Cranberry Detox Drink

4 tbsp of pure Organic unsweetened Cranberry Juice
2 tbsp of pure Organic Lemon Juice
1 tbsp of Organic Apple cider vinegar
8 oz of filtered water

I usually mix a big bottle of the ingredients 4:2:1 and keep it in the fridge. That way it is easy every morning to mix 3.5 oz of detox mix with 8 oz of filtered water.

Dry Brushing

Dry brushing is a Simple Detox Tool that demands just five minutes of your day, costs only the initial investment in a quality brush, and offers profound benefits for both the inner and outer health of your body.

Your skin, being the body's largest organ, plays a vital role in toxin elimination and nutrient absorption, making its health and functionality crucial to your overall well-being.

The skin's ability to absorb substances is indeed impressive. Research suggests that up to 60% of certain compounds applied to the skin can be absorbed. This highlights the importance of being mindful about what you apply to your skin, as it can have a significant impact on your health.

Also it is known that anything applied to or put on your skin can enter your bloodstream within as little as 26 seconds. This highlights the skin's efficiency as a gateway, and why it is so important to take good care of it.

On the other hand, around one-third of your body's toxins are expelled through the skin, underscoring the skin's essential role in the body's detox processes.

This natural mechanism relies on the effective functioning of your skin's pores and its ability to eliminate waste and harmful toxins. However, when your pores become clogged, this natural detoxification process is hindered, allowing toxins to accumulate within the skin.

Therefore, maintaining the health and vitality of your skin is not only crucial for its appearance but also for supporting your overall well-being and detox capabilities.

Here's a deeper look at why and how your skin acts as this pivotal interface:

Toxin Elimination

Your skin is equipped with countless tiny pores that release sweat and other bodily fluids. These fluids carry waste products and toxins from your body's deeper layers to the surface. When your pores are clear and unobstructed, this natural detoxification process operates smoothly, allowing toxins to exit the body efficiently through perspiration.
However, when pores become clogged due to factors like excess sebum production or the accumulation of dead skin cells, this vital elimination pathway is compromised. As a result, toxins may become trapped within the skin, potentially leading to various skin issues and even systemic health concerns.

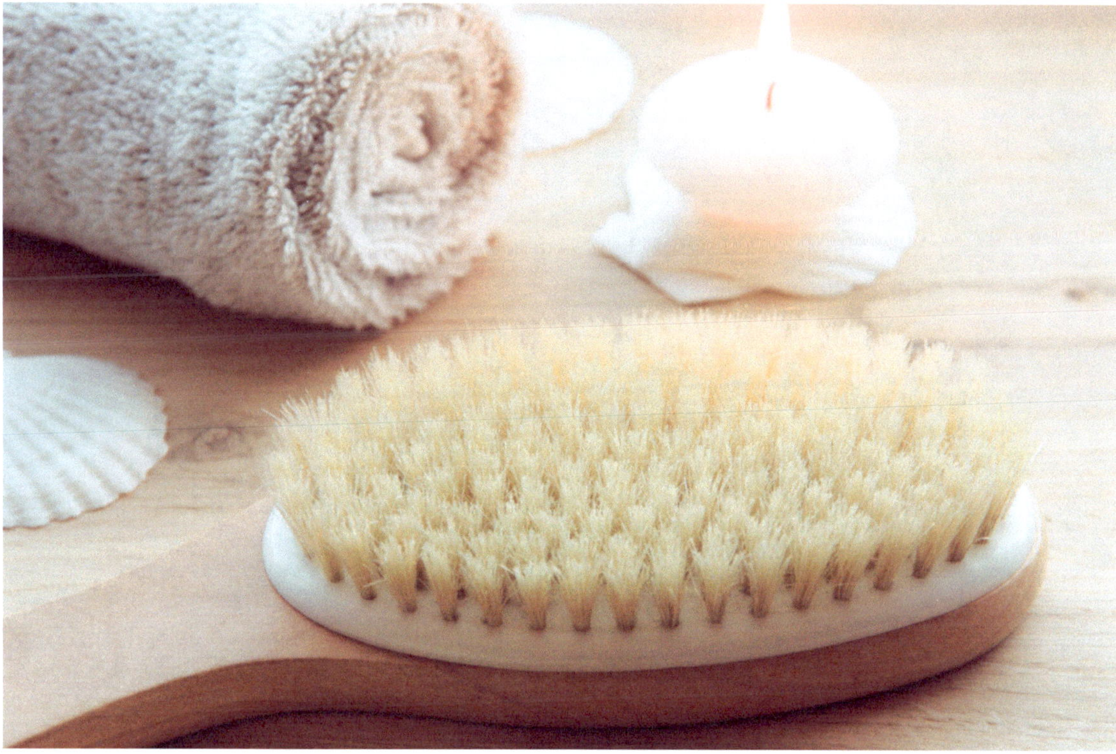

Nutrient Absorption

Just as your skin plays a role in eliminating waste, it also absorbs nutrients and beneficial substances.

The skin is not an impermeable barrier; instead, it allows certain substances to pass through its layers and enter the bloodstream. This is extremely relevant when applying topical treatments, such as skincare products or medications. The skin can absorb essential vitamins, minerals, and therapeutic compounds, enhancing their effectiveness in addressing various skin and health conditions.

Given the skin's dual role as both a detox and absorption pathway, it's vital to maintain its health and vitality. Practices like dry brushing, exfoliation, and proper skincare routines can help keep your pores clear and optimize toxin elimination.

Additionally, being mindful of the products you apply to your skin ensures that you benefit from nutrient absorption while avoiding potentially harmful substances.
By nurturing your skin's well-being, you support not only its radiant appearance but also your overall health and detoxification processes.

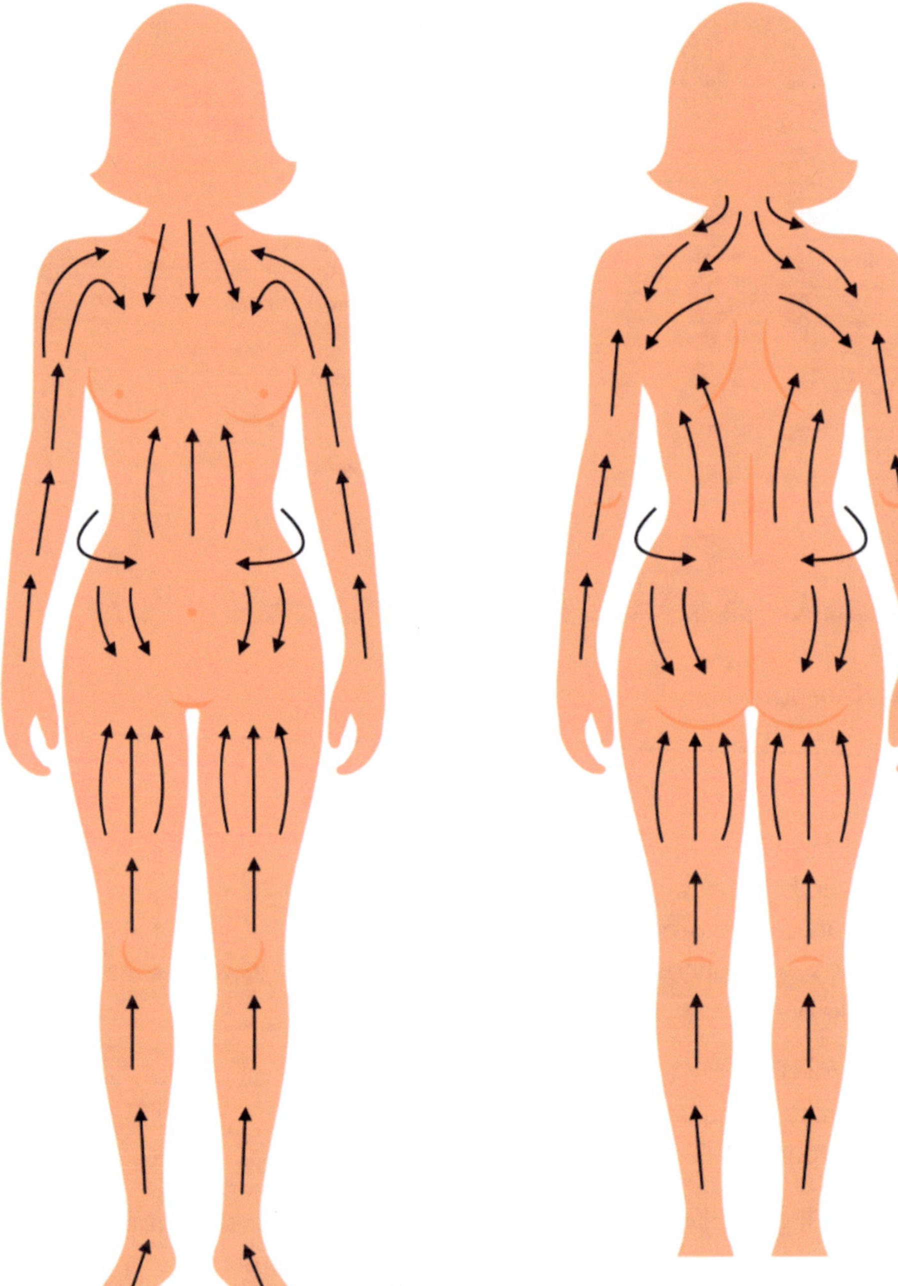

How To Dry Brush

1. To start, invest in a natural bristle brush with an extended handle to reach all areas of your body.
2. Stand in a bathtub, shower or on a tiled surface (while undressed) to catch the exfoliated skin.
3. Begin brushing from your feet, moving in long sweeping motions toward your heart, ensuring that you always brush in this direction. Be gentle when brushing over sensitive areas like your breasts; your skin will gradually become less sensitive with regular dry brushing.
4. After completing your entire body, step into the shower and alternate between the hottest and coldest water temperatures you can tolerate. This encourages blood circulation, promoting healthier skin.
5. Pat your skin dry and apply a natural oil such as almond oil or coconut oil.

For optimal results, do the Dry Brushing every day (twice a day is even better).

Remember to clean your brush with soap and water weekly and let it air dry in a clean, sunny spot to prevent mildew buildup. Try this transformative practice for 30 days, and witness the remarkable improvements in your skin's texture, detoxification process, and overall well-being.

Find the How To Dry Brush illustration on www.mygoodwitch.com/bookresources

Why Dry Brush

Dry brushing supports an array of health advantages that extend beyond the ones mentioned earlier.

Exfoliation

It effectively removes dead skin cells, leaving your skin consistently smooth and radiant throughout the year.

Lymphatic Stimulation

Dry brushing stimulates the lymphatic system, which acts as a drainage network for toxins in your body. This helps in the efficient removal of waste and harmful substances.

Cellulite Reduction

By breaking down and releasing toxic materials trapped in your body's fat cells, dry brushing may help reduce the appearance of cellulite.

Unclogged Pores

It unclogs and clears your pores, allowing your skin to breathe and better absorb essential nutrients.

Stress Reduction

The gentle pressure and rhythmic motion of dry brushing can have a calming effect on the nervous system, reducing stress and promoting relaxation.

Improved Circulation

Dry brushing enhances blood circulation, which can contribute to overall cardiovascular health and better oxygenation of tissues.

Cell Renewal

The removal of dead skin cells through dry brushing can promote cell turnover, leading to a more youthful and glowing complexion.

Enhanced Immune Function

A stimulated lymphatic system can support your immune response, potentially helping your body ward off infections more effectively.

Skin Tone and Texture

Consistent dry brushing can lead to improved skin tone, texture, and elasticity, helping you achieve healthier-looking skin.

So you see why incorporating dry brushing into your daily routine plays an important role in both your physical and mental well-being.

Foot Baths

Detox foot baths can offer a unique combination of potential toxin removal and relaxation. The warm water, herbal infusions, or salts used in these baths can promote relaxation by helping to ease tension and reduce stress, as well as helping pull out toxins and other waste from your body.

Even though the effectiveness of Detox Foot Baths is a subject of debate within the scientific community, most people find them relaxing and very beneficial.

Some of my favorite Detox Foot Baths are Ionic-, Essential Oil- and Epsom Salt Foot Baths, and I try to do them as often as possible.

Ionic Foot Baths

The ionic foot bath is based on the bioenergetics technology that creates an energy field similar to the human body's. The principal is similar to how a magnet works, except in this case the magnetic force functions to help cancel out and eliminate harmful free radicals and other toxins from the body.

Throughout the process, the water in the bath can change color, and you may observe tiny, colored flecks floating within it. This is due to toxins and waste materials being removed from your body.

Some of the benefits of an Ionic Foot Bath are:

enhanced lymph circulation, increased energy levels, decreased inflammation, migraine and headache relief, improved sleep quality, increased relaxation, support for the immune system in fighting off viruses, relief from muscle and joint pain, and reduced swelling

If you don't want to invest in a Ionic foot bath yourself, you can most likely find a health practitioner near you who offers sessions.

Essential Oil Foot Baths

Essential oils are highly concentrated extracts derived from plants, such as flowers, leaves, bark, stems, and roots. They are known for their aromatic properties and have been used for centuries in traditional medicine, perfumery, and various therapeutic practices.

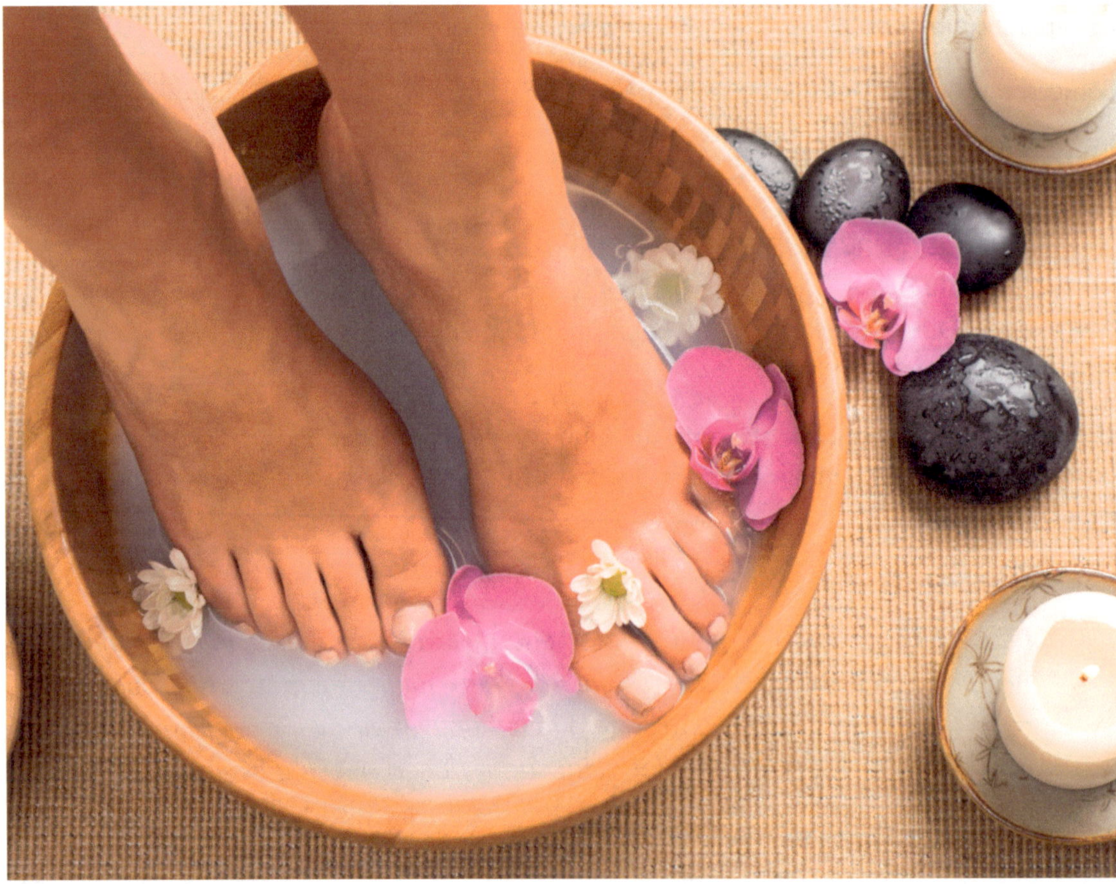

An essential oil foot bath offers a range of benefits, including relaxation detox, depending on the oils used. Some of the benefits of an essential oil foot bath are:

relaxation, improved sleep, detox, reduced stress,
anxiety relief, pain relief, and skin care

Essential oils like lavender, chamomile, and ylang-ylang are known for their relaxing properties. Soaking your feet in a foot bath with these oils can help reduce stress, anxiety, and promote an overall sense of calm and well-being.

When it comes to Detox, my favorite essential oils for Detox Foot Baths are:

Lemon supports lymphatic drainage and boosts your energy.

Grapefruit supports the lymphatic system, helps with fluid retention and toxin elimination.

Juniper Berry removes waste and toxins from the body, and has soothing effects on muscles and joints.

Lavender for relaxation and improved sleep

I can highly recommend finding an Essential Oil distributor who can teach you all the amazing ways you can use them.

This is what you need for an Essential Oil Foot Bath:

1 Foot Spa, or tub big enough for your feet
2 drops of Lemon oil
2 drops of Grapefruit oil
2 drops of Juniper Berry oil
2 drops of Lavender oil

Warm water - enough to cover your ankles.
Soak your feet for 15-20 minutes, allowing the oils to work their magic.

You can use all oils in one foot bath or choose one or two.

Epsom Salt Foot Baths

Epsom salt, also known as magnesium sulfate, is a naturally occurring mineral compound consisting of magnesium, sulfur, and oxygen.

It derives its name from the town of Epsom in England, where it was first discovered in mineral springs. This natural compound has a longstanding history of use for its therapeutic properties, making it a trusted addition to foot baths for those seeking to unwind, revitalize, and potentially support their overall well-being

Incorporating Epsom salt into your foot baths offers a variety of health and therapeutic benefits. When dissolved in water, Epsom salt releases magnesium and sulfate ions that can be absorbed through the skin, contributing to soothing and revitalizing effects making it a go-to solution for soothing tired feet and promoting relaxation.

Some of the best known benefits of using Epsom Salt in your Detox Foot Bath are:

muscle relaxation, detox, stress reduction, improved sleep,
reduced inflammation, pain relief, and improved circulation.

If you don't already have Epsom Salt in your cabinet, you should definitely buy some and start treating yourself to a calming Detox Foot Bath on a regular basis.

This is what you need for an Epsom Salt Foot Bath:

1 Foot Spa, or tub big enough for your feet
1/2 cup of Epsom Salt

Warm water - enough to cover your ankles.
Soak your feet for 15-20 minutes, allowing the oils to work their magic.
I like to add 2 drops of lavender oil to mine as well.

Supplements, Herbs And Plants

Incorporating supplements into your detox regimen can be beneficial because they can provide targeted support to enhance the body's natural detoxification processes.

Our bodies are designed to eliminate toxins on its own, but as you know by now, modern diets and lifestyles don't always provide the necessary nutrients and in sufficient quantities to support this natural process of detox.

Adding supplements like activated charcoal, chlorella, vitamin C and glutathione as well as herbs such as milk thistle and dandelion root, all offer great support when it comes to helping the body detox from pollutants, heavy metals, and harmful substances.

Before you start buying all the supplements, make sure to consult a Holistic Health Practitioner. There are so many other supplements for detox support our there than the ones mentioned in this section, and you need to know which ones are good for you. Also, you may only need one or two, or maybe none at all.

Find my favorites through www.mygoodwitch.com/bookresources

Activated Charcoal

Activated charcoal is derived from carbon-rich sources like coconut shells or wood, and are processed to become highly porous. Their unique structure allows them to bind to toxins and chemicals in the digestive tract, preventing their absorption into the body.

This makes activated charcoal a popular choice for detoxification, as it acts like a sponge, aiding in the removal of unwanted substances.

Some of the benefits of using Activated Charcoal for detoxifying are:

improved digestion, reduced gas and bloating, improved liver function and skin health, as well as reduced heavy metal poisoning.

Chlorella

Chlorella is a type of green algae that is another great supplement when it comes to detox. It has high levels of chlorophyll, antioxidants, essential amino acids, vitamin A, C and K, as well as iron, magnesium and potassium. It is also a great source of fibers.

Some of the potential benefits of using chlorella supplements are:

improved digestion, skin health, liver- & immune function,
as well as lower the risk of oxidative stress and chronic diseases.

Vitamin C

Vitamin C, also known as ascorbic acid, is a water-soluble vitamin that plays a crucial role in various physiological processes within the human body. It is an essential nutrient, meaning the body cannot produce it on its own, you must have it through your diet, or as a supplement.

As an antioxidant, vitamin C can neutralize free radicals and support the body's natural detox processes. It's also essential for the production of glutathione

Some of the benefits of Vitamin C are:

immune support, decrease stress, support collagen production,
supports heart health, and cognitive function

Glutathione

Glutathione is a powerful antioxidant and a tripeptide made from three amino acids: cysteine, glutamic acid, and glycine., and is naturally produced in the body.

However, a number of factors such as aging, chronic illnesses, and environmental toxins, can deplete glutathione levels. In such cases, supplementation with glutathione or its precursors (such as N-acetylcysteine or a good quality whey protein) should be considered.

Glutathione is known to be good for:

cellular repair, skin health, respiratory health, neurological health, liver support,
lower inflammation, and support for other antioxidants like Vitamin C and E

Cilantro

Also known as coriander, cilantro is a highly adaptable herb that offers numerous health benefits. It contains a variety of essential nutrients and compounds that support detoxification. Cilantro is an excellent source of vitamin C and K, which are essential for bone health and immune support. It also provides important minerals like potassium, calcium, manganese, and iron. These minerals play important role in regulating

blood pressure, maintaining bone strength, and supporting various bodily functions.

Additionally, cilantro is high in phytonutrients and flavonoids which are very anti-inflammatory, as well as antioxidants, such as beta-carotene, quercetin, and rutin, which help combat

oxidative stress and reduce the risk of chronic diseases.

Cilantro is especially great when it comes to removal of heavy metals from the body as well as reducing digestive discomfort.

If you use cilantro microgreens you get the most nutritional value and you can use a handful as topping on tacos, salads, salsas, chicken, pasta dishes and asian dishes.

Milk Thistle

Milk thistle is well known for its exceptional support to the liver. Its active compound, silymarin, plays a crucial role in optimal liver health and function. Silymarin acts as a protective shield for the liver, guarding it against the harmful toxins, pollutants, and even certain medications. By reducing oxidative stress and inflammation within the liver, milk thistle helps prevent damage to liver cells and tissues. Furthermore, silymarin supports the regeneration of liver cells, the liver's ability to repair itself and plays a vital role in the detox process.

You can get milk thistle as a tea which you can mix with the dandelion, or you can get it in a capsule, and use it 30 days every quarter, or as needed.

Dandelion

Another great plant to use is Dandelion. It is best known as a weed, but make no mistake, Dandelion is a powerhouse of essential nutrients, including vitamins A, C, and K, as well as minerals like iron, calcium, and potassium. Beyond its nutritional value, dandelion is well known when it comes to detox. It acts as a natural diuretic, supporting increased urine production and helping flush toxins from the body.

Dandelion's detox effect is especially used for the liver and gallbladder, where it supports the efficient processing and elimination of waste and toxins. Its high antioxidant content also helps fight oxidative stress and inflammation.

As for the milk thistle, you can get dandelion as tea or in capsules, and I will suggest you use both milk thistle and dandelion together for maximum detox support.

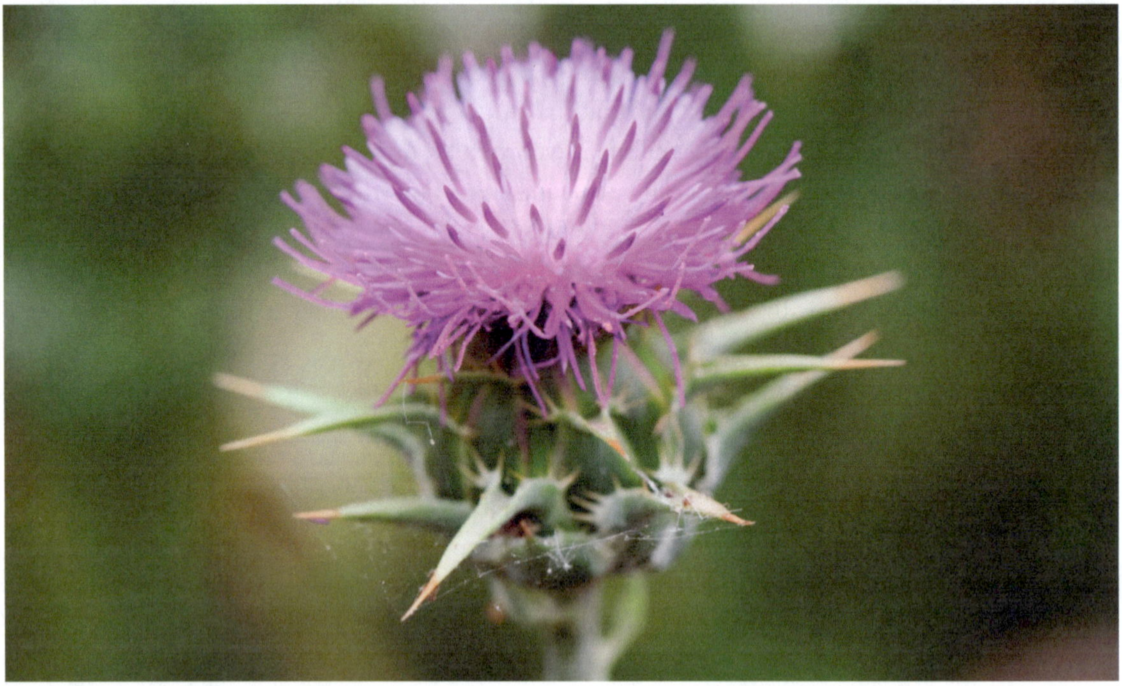

Healthy Living

These were just some of my favorite simple detox tools, which are all something that is easy to incorporate without investing a lot of money, yet still get the maximum outcome of your efforts.

Whether through *Simple Detox Tools like supplements, oil pulling, detox drinks, foot baths, or dry brushing, you have the opportunity to support your body's natural cleansing processes, reduce symptoms and develop a renewed sense of vitality. As you remove harmful toxins, reduce inflammation, and promote overall health, you may find that the path to a healthier, more vibrant life becomes clearer and more attainable. Remember, while these tools can be valuable additions to your routine, they work best in conjunction with a mindful lifestyle and a mindful diet.

Disclaimer

**It is important to note that the use of the previously mentioned simple detox tools should be done under the guidance of a healthcare professional, as it can interact with certain medications and can have adverse effects if used improperly.*

Chapter Thirteen

STRESS MANAGEMENT

Stress Management means taking control of various aspects of your life, such as your lifestyle, thoughts, emotions, and problem-solving methods. No matter how overwhelming life may seem, there are steps you can take to alleviate stress and regain a sense of control. We all know that life can get overwhelming. The bills keep coming, you don't have enough hours in a day and your responsibilities both at work and at home keep piling up. It feels like there's nothing you can do about it. I beg to differ. You have more control over it than you might think.

It is crucial to understand that stress is not the same as simply being busy. Although being too busy for too long, conscious or subconscious, might create stress over time.

Also your surroundings play a huge role in your stress levels. Constant noise, excessive light, persistent Wi-Fi signals, TV, and continuous music can contribute to keeping our bodies in a state resembling the "fight or flight" response associated with stress. These environmental factors can overstimulate our senses, triggering the release of stress hormones like cortisol and adrenaline.

Constant exposure to lots of sounds, lights, and activities can mess up our body's natural rhythms, making it hard to relax and fully rest. This can cause long-term stress, sleep problems, and health issues. It's very important that we set up spaces where we can have peaceful moments and give our senses a break. This helps balance out the impact of our busy and overstimulated lifestyles. (Go back to My Seven Steps, Silence, in chapter eight).

To create a calm and sensory restful environment, consider making some simple changes. Start by minimizing loud noises and bright lights in your space, especially during the evening. Create a comfortable and cozy atmosphere with soft lighting and soothing colors. Incorporate elements like plants or nature-inspired decor to bring a sense of calm. Additionally, practice activities that promote relaxation, such as gentle stretching, deep breathing, or listening to calming music. By making these adjustments, you can enhance your environment and support a healthier balance for your body and mind.

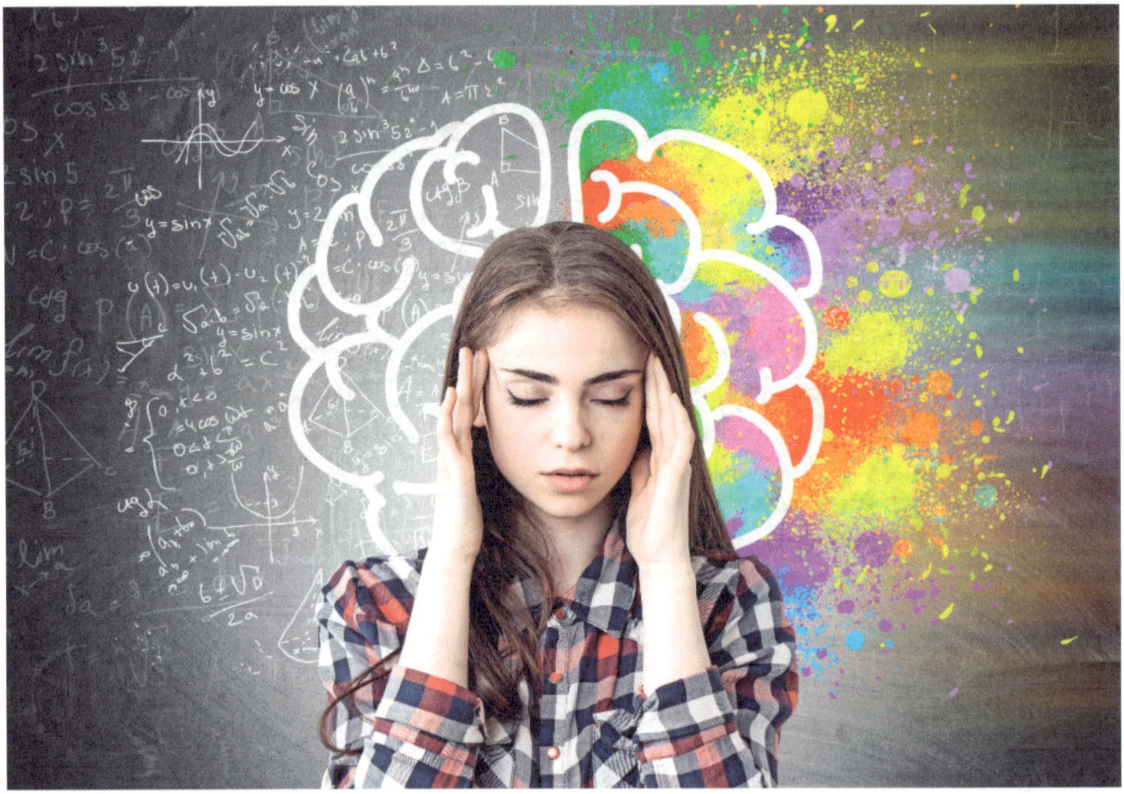

Understanding the significance of stress management is crucial. High levels of stress can jeopardize your overall well-being. It disrupts your emotional balance and has a negative impact on your physical health, impairing your ability to think clearly, function effectively, and find joy in life.

On the contrary, effective stress management empowers you to break free from the grip of stress, leading to a happier, healthier, and more productive life. The ultimate aim is to achieve a balanced life that includes time for work, relationships, relaxation, and enjoyment, while also building resilience to face challenges with confidence.

Our lives are filled with things to do –
Family, friends, and jobs all need our attention.
Too often you forget about YOU!

~Birgitte Haaning Christensen

Dealing with stress isn't the same for everyone, and unfortunately there's no magic solution that fits everyone perfectly. That's why it's super important to try out different things and figure out what helps you the most. What works for one person might not work for another, so be patient and kind to yourself as you explore different stress management strategies.

Understand Stress

High stress levels can harm your emotional balance and physical health, making it challenging to think clearly, be effective, or enjoy life. Effective stress management is key to breaking free from stress's grip and leading a balanced life with time for work, relationships, relaxation, and fun.

To manage stress, start by identifying its sources, which may not always be obvious. Reflect on your habits, attitudes, and excuses, and recognize your role in creating stress. Keeping a stress journal can be helpful, allowing you to note what's causing stress, how it makes you feel, and your reactions, revealing patterns and enhancing your understanding.

Both unconscious and conscious stress can significantly impact your health. Unconscious stress, often lingering beneath awareness, can manifest in physical and emotional symptoms, such as headaches, muscle tension, irritability, and weakened immunity. It's crucial to pay attention to subtle signs and address them early through self-check-ins, mindfulness practices, and stress management techniques. Similarly, conscious stress, when recognized, may lead to persistent worry, tension, and physical manifestations like elevated blood pressure or disrupted sleep.

Adopting healthy coping mechanisms, seeking support, and practicing stress-reducing activities are essential in eliminating the negative effects of conscious stress on your overall well-being.

Take Control

Taking control and recognizing stress is the starting point for effective stress management. It's about understanding that you have the power to navigate various aspects of your life, forming the foundation to steer through stress.

Exerting command over your lifestyle, thoughts, emotions, and problem-solving approaches is essential. Remember, no matter how tough life gets, there are practical steps within your reach to ease stress.

In addition to embracing this sense of control, developing self-awareness is key. Regularly check in with yourself, pinpoint stress triggers, and understand how your body and mind react. This heightened awareness enhances your ability to proactively manage stress, allowing you to implement strategies tailored to your unique needs. (See chapter eleven, Self Awareness.

Create Healthy Habits

Look at your current lifestyle and how you deal with conscious stress. Are you promoting good health, or could you benefit from some improvement?

Habits such as smoking, excessive drinking, overeating, inactivity or procrastinating can all contribute to stress. Therefore it is essential to exchange these habits for healthier ones that contribute to your overall well-being.

Engaging in activities like regular exercise, mindful living, and maintaining mindful eating, not only supports physical health but also plays a significant role in your mental health and will reduce or eliminate stress. Incorporating these healthy habits, you are not only investing long term in your well-being, you are also creating a healthy mental balance against stress.

It Is Ok To Say No

Stress is a natural response triggered by your nervous system, and some stressors follow predictable patterns, like your daily commute, certain meetings, tasks or family gatherings. When dealing with these known stressors, you have two options: change the situation or adapt your response.

While it's not advisable to avoid challenging situations that require your attention, you might be surprised by the number of stressors in your life that can be eliminated. Develop the skill of saying "no" by understanding your limits and respecting them, whether in your personal or professional life.

Taking on more than you can handle is a sure path to stress, so differentiate between tasks you "should" do and those you "must" do. Whenever possible, decline tasks that exceed your capacity. If specific individuals consistently contribute to your stress, consider limiting your time with them or let go of the relationship all together.

Recognizing your limits and learning the power of saying no is an essential aspect of stress management. Saying no and setting boundaries is not a sign of weakness but a conscious choice for self-care, and you empower yourself to navigate stress effectively. This simple yet powerful practice of saying no, creates a more sustainable and balanced lifestyle, enabling you to better manage the demands of daily life.

Additionally, take charge of your surroundings by minimizing exposure to stressors, such as anxiety-inducing news outlets and social media. When facing traffic stress, choose a less-traveled route if possible. If grocery shopping feels like a daunting chore, explore online alternatives or pay someone to do it for you. Simplify your to-do list by evaluating your schedule, responsibilities, and daily tasks. If you find yourself overwhelmed, prioritize essential tasks and either postpone or eliminate the non-essential ones.

When avoiding stress isn't an option, focus on changing the situation by modifying how you communicate and navigate your daily life. Practice how to express your emotions rather than keeping them bottled up. If something or someone is causing you distress, you have to share your concerns openly and respectfully. Failing to voice your feelings can lead to resentment and increased stress levels.

Be active

Exercise is a fantastic stress reliever. It releases feel-good chemicals in your brain and helps distract you from worries. You don't need to be a gym fanatic. Just get moving by dancing, walking, riding your bike or doing activities you enjoy. Also consider relaxation practices like yoga, meditation, grounding and deep breathing to calm your mind and body, and keep you balanced.

Don't forget to take care of YOU. Schedule "me" time in your day for activities you enjoy, like stargazing, playing music, or relaxing in a warm bath. A sense of humor also helps fight stress.

Spending time with people who make you feel safe and understood is incredibly calming. Face-to-face interactions trigger natural stress relief. Build and maintain connections with family and friends, even if they can't solve your problems. Simply having someone to talk to can make a big difference.

Time Management

Effective time management plays a very important role in your daily lives, productivity, success, and overall well-being. It is linked with stress management by the way you allocate and utilize your time, and can significantly impact your stress levels.

In the modern, fast-paced world, where demands and responsibilities seem to be constantly increasing, managing your time becomes essential for maintaining a healthy work-life balance and minimizing stressors. Knowing how to handle your time and stress is crucial. It's all about figuring out the best ways to prioritize tasks, set achievable goals, and make a schedule that works for you. Managing your time and being organized doesn't just help you get more done – it's also a great way to deal with stress. By having a well-thought-out approach to your time, you not only boost productivity but also use it as a strong tool to lessen the negative impact of stress.

Work smarter, not harder

Do you ever feel like there's not enough time in the day? We all get the same 24 hours – so why do some people seem to achieve more with their time than others?
The answer: ***good time management.***

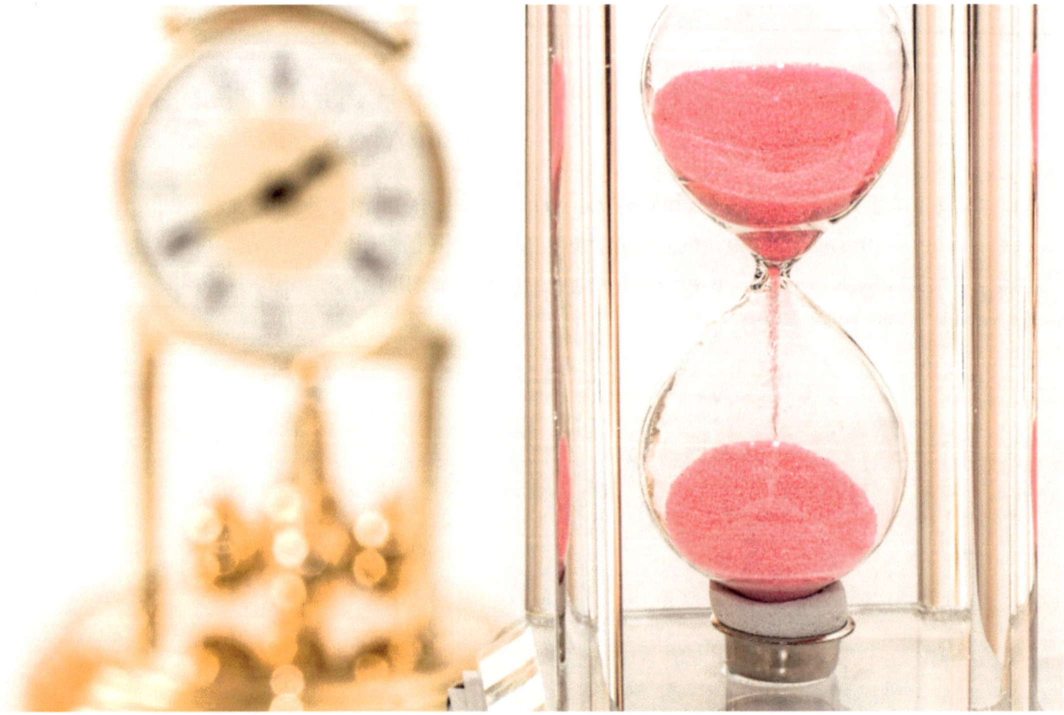

Time management is the process of organizing and planning how to divide your time between different activities. Get it right, and you'll end up working smarter, not harder, and get more done in less time – even when time is tight and pressures are high. The highest achievers manage their time exceptionally well.

Benefits Of Good Time Management

Time management is a fundamental skill that will positively impact various aspects of your live. Proper time management allows you to make the most out of your day both in your professional and your personal life. By prioritizing tasks and setting realistic goals, you can accomplish more in less time. This not only increases productivity but also provides a sense of accomplishment.

Your stress level will also go down because, when you plan your days efficiently, you are better equipped to handle challenges, unexpected events, and deadlines. This proactive mindset reduces the pressure you feel and contributes to a healthier work-life balance.

Another benefit is that when you allocate specific time slots for different tasks based on their importance and urgency, you improve your ability to focus. This increased focused attention leads to better-quality work and a more efficient use of your mental energy.

Overall, you'll start feeling more in control with the confidence to choose how best to use your time. And by feeling happier, more relaxed, and better able to think, you're in a great place to help others reach their goals too.

How well do you manage your time?

Start by assessing your existing approach. How good are you at organizing your time so that you get the important things done well? Can you balance your time between different activities? And when you do make time to do something, are you able to focus – and get it finished?

Tip: Good time management takes a shift in focus from activities to results. Being busy isn't the same as being effective. In fact, for many people, the busier they are, the less they actually achieve.

"If you fail to plan, you are planning to fail!"

~Benjamin Franklin

Stress And Time Management Tools

You now know the importance of managing your time and stress, and how they can affect your well being if you don't.

Here are my top 10 tips on how to have better stress and time management:

To-Do Lists

Create a list of tasks you need to complete, prioritizing them by importance and deadlines.

To-do lists offer a multitude of benefits for personal and professional productivity. They provide a structured and organized approach to managing tasks, allowing you to prioritize your responsibilities by importance and deadlines. Tools like paper planners, digital apps, or simple handwritten lists can be used to help you keep track. By breaking down large goals into smaller, actionable items, to-do lists facilitate progress and goal achievement.

They reduce stress and mental clutter by externalizing tasks from memory, leading to increased focus and reduced anxiety. They also promote effective time management, making sure that valuable time is spent on high-priority tasks, as well as offering flexibility for adapting to changing circumstances.

Last but not least, crossing something off the list fills you with a sense of accomplishment, motivation and accountability, which ultimately leads to success and productivity in other aspects of your life.

Time Blocking

Allocating specific blocks of time for different tasks or activities, offers several notable benefits for personal and professional productivity.

It prevents procrastination by establishing a specific start time for each activity, reducing the likelihood of delaying tasks. When tasks are scheduled and time-bound, it becomes easier to track progress, assess productivity, and make adjustments as needed.

Also, it helps you focus and concentrate by encouraging you to devote your full attention to a single task during a designated time period, reducing the urge to multitask, which can lead to decreased efficiency and increased stress.

By scheduling tasks and activities, you create a clear plan for your day, ensuring that essential responsibilities are addressed and that time is used purposefully. This approach also helps you estimate how much time various tasks require, making it easier to set realistic goals and deadlines. Using a specific time to high-priority items, ensures you that critical work gets the attention it deserves.

One of my favorite benefits of time blocking is having a healthy work-life balance by setting boundaries and ensuring that time is allocated for personal and leisure activities. This can help prevent burnout and maintain overall well-being.

Goal Setting

Setting goals is a fundamental practice that brings numerous advantages to both personal and professional life. By clearly defining your short-term and long-term goals, you create a structured and purposeful path forward. This clarity not only provides you with a sense of direction but also helps you use your time and resources more effectively, as you can focus on activities and tasks that directly contribute to achieving those goals.

Goals also serve as powerful motivators. When you have well-defined objectives, you are more likely to stay committed and persistent in the face of challenges. They give you a reason to push beyond your comfort zone, learn new skills, and adapt to changing circumstances, ultimately fostering personal growth and development.

Also, setting goals enhances decision-making. With a clear understanding of what you want to achieve, you can make informed choices that align with your aspirations. This reduces the likelihood of getting sidetracked by distractions or unrelated activities, as you are more likely to prioritize tasks that bring you closer to your goals.

Furthermore, goal setting gives a sense of accountability. You can track your progress, celebrate small victories along the way, and adjust your strategies if you encounter obstacles. This ongoing feedback loop ensures that you are continually improving and moving closer to your desired outcomes.

Lastly, goal setting is a powerful tool that provides direction, motivation, and at the same time improves your time management, decision-making, and accountability. It empowers you to pursue their dreams with purpose and determination, leading to greater fulfillment and success in various aspects of life.

Mind Mapping

Mind mapping is a way to show information visually. It's like drawing a tree with a main idea in the middle and smaller ideas connected to it like branches. This helps you organize thoughts, ideas, or plans in a simple and clear way. It allows you to break down complex topics or projects into smaller, manageable components, making it easier to structure your thoughts and prioritize tasks. You can use pictures or short words to represent each idea, making it easier to understand complex topics.

It is also great for brainstorming, planning projects and enhancing creativity. It encourages free-flowing, non-linear thinking, making it easier to generate new ideas, associations, and solutions. The visual format of mind maps can spark creative insights and facilitate innovative problem-solving, helps you see the bigger picture and organize your thoughts. And improve information retention. When you engage both the visual and spatial aspects of your brain, you create a more memorable mental representation of the information. This can aid in recalling details and concepts more effectively.

Transforming mind mapping into a fun project can be both engaging and productive. Use colorful pens or digital tools to create visually appealing mind maps, and don't be afraid to get creative with drawings, icons, or even stickers to represent ideas. Challenge yourself to connect concepts in unique and unexpected ways, turning the process into a playful exercise of imagination. By adding fun and creativity into mind mapping, you can make learning and organizing information an exciting and rewarding experience.

Saying No

Just as we went through in the Stress management section, saying no is a crucial skill in both personal and professional life, because it enables you to maintain a sense of balance and control over your time and energy. When you politely decline commitments and tasks that don't align with your goals or values, you ensure that your resources are directed toward what truly matters to you. This means you can invest more time in activities that contribute to your personal growth, well-being, and long-term objectives.

Overcommitting, on the other hand, can lead to a host of issues. It can strain your time management capabilities, leaving you feeling overwhelmed and stretched thin. You might find it challenging to meet deadlines or perform tasks effectively when your plate is overly full. This will, over time, result in increased stress levels and a decreased quality of work.

Furthermore, constantly saying yes to every request can undermine your own priorities and aspirations. You might end up neglecting your personal and professional development because you're too busy fulfilling others' demands.

Learning to say no allows you to set boundaries, protect your time, and ensure that you're making choices in alignment with your values and long-term goals.

In essence, mastering the art of saying no is a powerful skill that fosters better time management, reduces stress, and ensures that your actions are congruent with your values and objectives. It's a vital component of maintaining a healthy work-life balance and achieving long-term success and fulfillment.

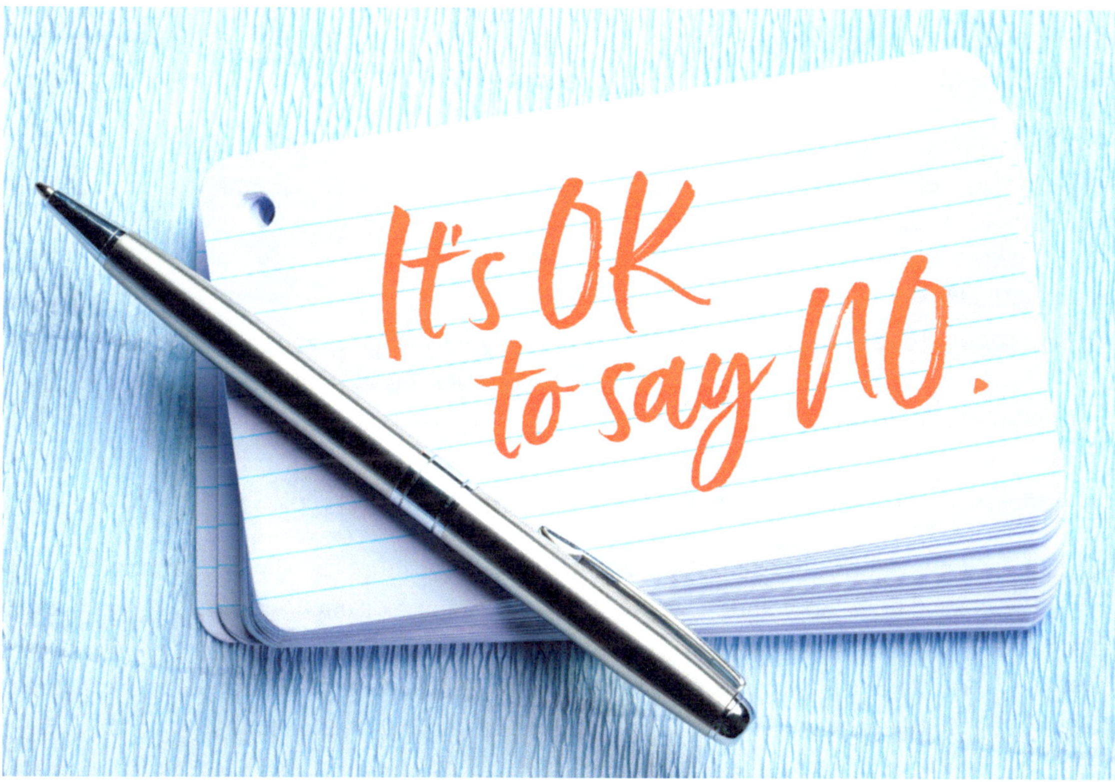

Self-Care

Self-care plays a pivotal role in effective stress and time management because it directly impacts your overall productivity and well-being. When you make time for self-care activities like exercise, meditation, and relaxation, you're investing in your mental and physical health. A well-rested and healthy mind is not only more alert and focused but also capable of making better decisions and managing time more efficiently.

Engaging in regular exercise, for instance, boosts energy levels, reduces stress, and enhances mental clarity, all of which contribute to better time management. Similarly, meditation and relaxation techniques can help you manage stress, improve concentration, and enhance your ability to prioritize tasks.

Also, self-care activities offer a break from the demands of a busy schedule, providing an opportunity to recharge and rejuvenate. This, in turn, can prevent burnout and increase your resilience in the face of challenging tasks or tight deadlines.

Therefore, integrating self-care into your time management routine is crucial because it ensures that you're operating at your best, and helps you to a better overall time management and work-life balance.

Eliminate Distractions

You might not think much of this, but distractions directly impact your ability to stay focused and manage your time effectively. Identifying the distractions in your environment and taking steps to minimize them is a key strategy for enhancing productivity. When you recognize and address distractions, such as notifications, irrelevant websites, or disorganized workspaces, you create a conducive environment for concentration and task completion.

Turning off notifications, for example, prevents interruptions that can divert your attention and disrupt your workflow. Apple and Google Watches are huge distractions whether you want to recognize it or not. Using website blockers helps you resist the temptation of mindlessly browsing the internet when you should be working. Creating a dedicated and organized workspace minimizes physical distractions and enhances your mental clarity.

By eliminating the above disruptions, you free up mental space to concentrate on essential tasks, improving your time management and overall productivity. This, in turn, allows you to work more efficiently and accomplish goals more effectively.

Delegate

This one is crucial both in professional and personal life. Delegating enables you to tap into the strengths and expertise of others, freeing up your time for more important activities. Whether at work or home, when you delegate you not only give responsibilities and a sense of ownership to coworkers or family members, you also give yourself the feeling of accomplishment. This allows you to focus on high-priority activities, and to be more efficient and productive both in your professional and personal life.

So, whether you're managing a team at work or delegating household chores among family members, the benefits of delegation extend to various aspects of life, leading to better time management and more success.

Continuous Improvement

Continuous improvement is not only essential for effective stress and time management but also for overall personal and professional growth. It keeps you in a mindset of learning and abundance you can use in all aspects of life. Embracing the idea that what works today might not work tomorrow encourages you always to learn new methods and strategies.

This commitment to continuous improvement enhances problem-solving skills, increases self-awareness, and gives you a sense of accomplishment, ultimately contributing to a more fulfilling and successful life. It enables you to navigate challenges, look for opportunities, and make consistent progress toward your goals, both in in your work life as well as personal life.

Don't be overwhelmed

The key to effective stress and time management is indeed finding the tools and techniques that work best for you and integrating them into your daily routine. Don't try to use all the tools I have mentioned at once. Start by picking one or two and incorporate them into your day. Once you master them, you can add more.

Your journey toward optimizing your time and minimizing your stress will likely involve some trial and error. It's essential to remember that what works for one person may not work for another, as everyone's work style, goals, and priorities differ. Embrace experimentation as a means of discovering your own stress and time management style. Be open to testing various strategies, tools, and workflows, and don't be afraid to adapt or customize them to suit your unique needs and goals.

Moreover, it's important to stay flexible and open-minded. As your responsibilities change, your life circumstances evolve, and new tools and technologies emerge, your stress and time management needs may shift as well.

Embrace continuous learning and improvement as part of your journey. Regularly assess your strategies, discard what no longer serves you, and embrace new approaches that better align with your current objectives.

Remember that effective stress and time management isn't just about doing more; it's about doing what matters most to you with focus and purpose. By staying committed to refining your steps and time management skills and staying attuned to your changing needs, you'll unlock the potential for greater productivity, reduced stress, and a more fulfilling life.

Declutter And Organize

Any time is a perfect time to declutter and organize. Many of us find ourselves spending more time at home, providing a golden opportunity to sift through the boxes and piles that have accumulated over the years. Holding onto unused items is akin to carrying around extra pounds or maintaining a negative state of mind.

Letting go of possessions that no longer serve a purpose creates not only physical space in your home but also a healthier mental state. The same principle applies to relationships that may have run their course. Despite the initial pain of saying goodbye to a person who was once a friend, the liberation felt afterward is immeasurable.

The health benefits of decluttering extend beyond mental and emotional well-being. Reduced anxiety, increased energy levels, enhanced confidence, and even a decrease in respiratory issues and allergies are among the positive outcomes. Clutter is a dust magnet, and by clearing it away, you create a cleaner and healthier living environment.

To tackle the decluttering process without skyrocketing stress levels, consider adopting a systematic approach. Start by scheduling dedicated time each day to work on one room, or break it down further into smaller areas like cabinets, drawers, or shelves. Discard clothes that no longer fit to avoid sending negative signals to your brain about body image. Letting go of possessions, much like shedding excess weight, is a powerful metaphor for personal growth.

For a more comprehensive decluttering experience, venture into storage spaces like under your bed or in the basement, attic, or garage. Recognize that emotional items stored under the bed may disrupt sleep patterns. If you need to use under-bed storage, limit it to items like blankets and pillows.

Address long-neglected boxes, like those containing old photos, and dedicate a focused weekend to the task. Involve your family, especially children, in the process. Not only will you make progress more efficiently, but you'll also share stories and memories associated with the items.

Soon you will embrace the lightness and sense of accomplishment that comes with decluttering and organizing your space. Remember, the process should be enjoyable and fulfilling. Have fun on this journey towards a more organized and harmonious living environment!

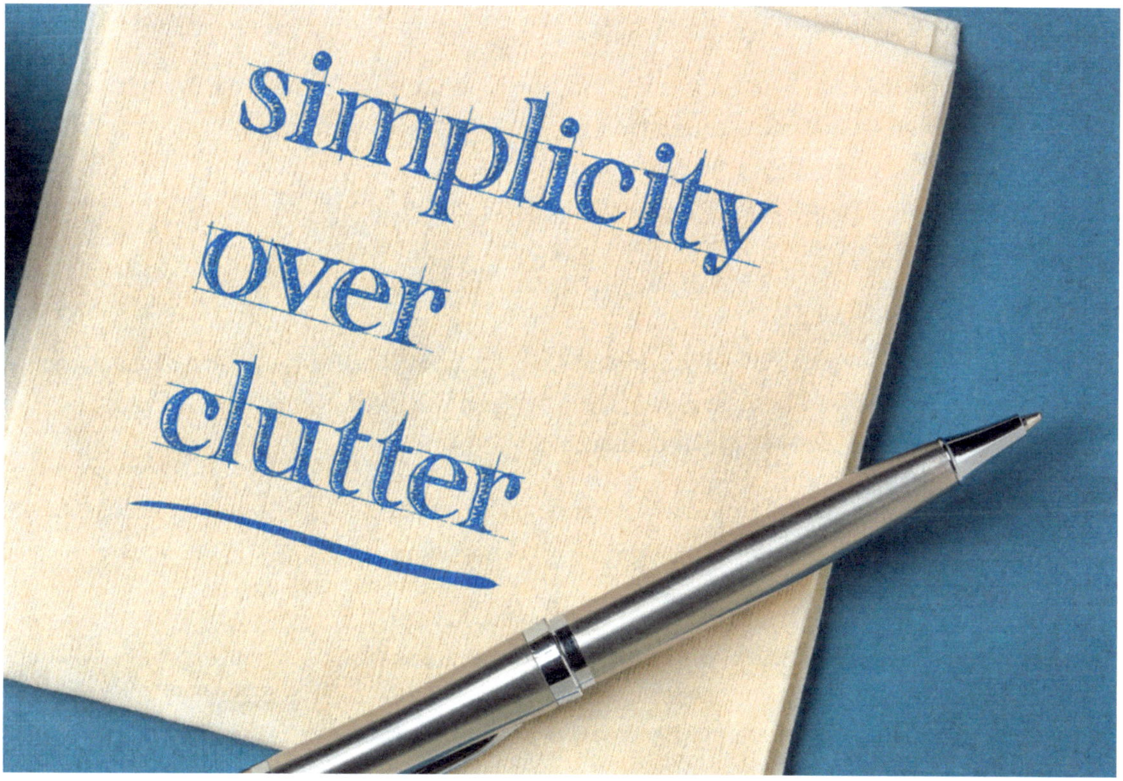

Silence

Silence is a very important part of your health and well-being. However, most people do not know what it means to be in, or have total silence. Fortunately it is very easy to learn.

Our fast paced modern world is full of background noise, music, tv's running, phones ringing, notifications coming in and people talking around you. This puts us in a constant fight and flight mode, which stresses your body tremendously.

Take a break twice a day when it fits into your daily routine.

Start with 5 minutes twice daily and work your way to at least 15 minutes twice daily.

Before you start your silence, I recommend you prepare your body and your brain, by doing 5 deep breaths. Then sit down in a quiet spot and just float away. You can use meditation, deep breaths exercises or just let your thoughts wander. As long as you don't get any noise from around you. You can also put on some soft music, or go for a walk in nature. Remember, the most important way of getting a great result is to do it and be consistent.

Why do we need silence?

By experiencing silence e.g. through meditation, you boost your self-esteem, motivation and joy. It gives you mental strength, and helps you let go of blocked energy. You will quickly gain increased awareness and get in better contact with yourself.

Silence will help you reflect on what has happened, recharge your batteries and help you relax, by freeing your mind from the constant stream of noise and stimuli you are surrounded with around the clock.

Because it lowers blood cortisol and adrenaline levels, the physiological benefits of silence include lower blood pressure, boosted immune system and brain chemistry, as well as stress reduction. Silence also helps you to be creative, realize your dreams, as well as discover who you are and how you feel.

Gratitude

Gratitude may be one of the most overlooked tools we have access to every day. It doesn't cost anything and doesn't take up much time, yet the benefits are enormous!
You show gratitude for what you receive, whether tangible or intangible. Meaning, you acknowledge the goodness in your life.

Gratitude is a great way to appreciate what you have instead of always reaching for a new shiny object, negativity or what you don't have. Although it may feel strange at first, this mental state grows stronger with use and practice.

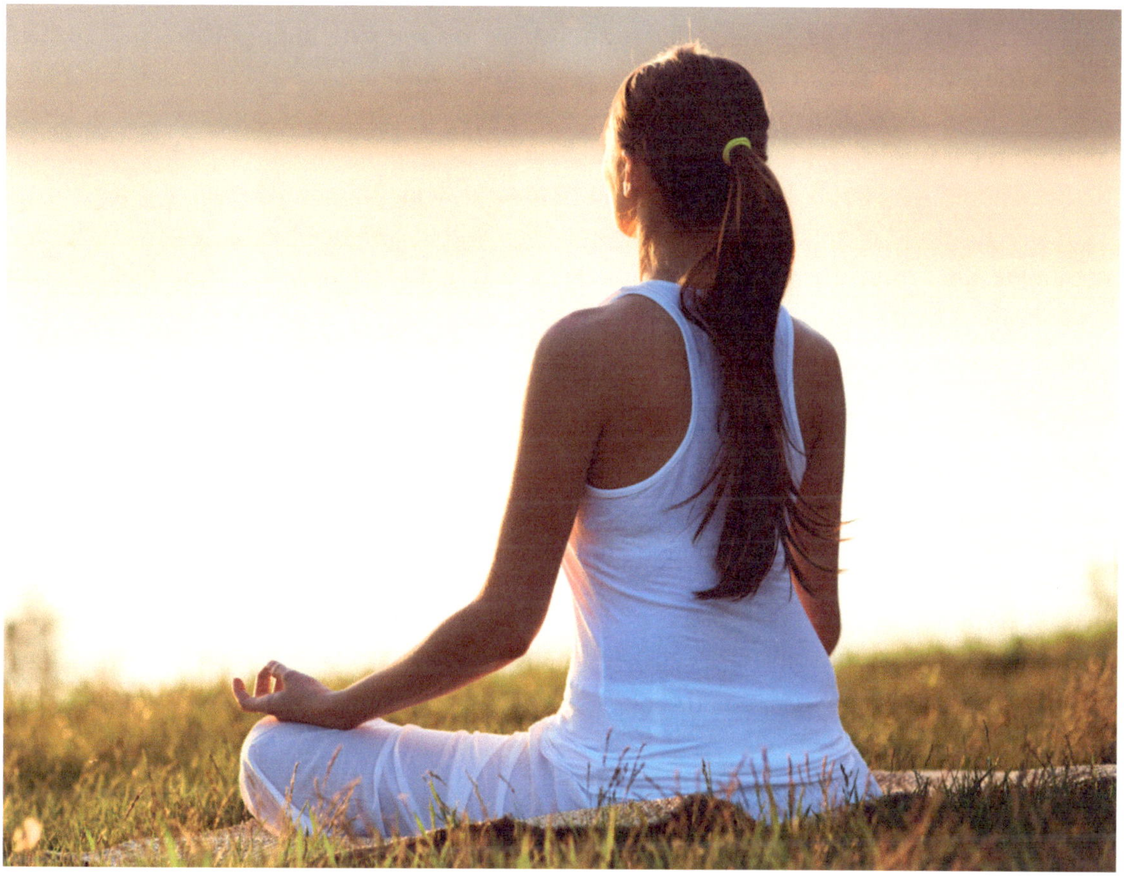

Too many focus on the negative and on what's wrong with their life, spouse, family, work and friends, and too little on all the good things in life i.e. waking up every day, having clothes to wear and food to eat.

Hearing the birds, getting a compliment, or a phone call from someone dear to you. Or maybe someone held the door for you at the store. It doesn't have to be huge events, but more recognizing the little things in life. As a result, being grateful also helps you connect to something larger than yourself as an individual - whether to other people, nature, or a higher power.

Gratitude is also associated with greater happiness, as it helps you feel more positive emotions, relish good experiences and improve your health.

Some of the benefits of having gratitude are:

Improves relationships

Gratitude opens the door to healthier relationships. By showing appreciation, saying thank you, holding the door for a stranger, or sending a thank you card to someone, you will attract new relationships which may lead to new opportunities. Studies show how gratitude can improve relationships. When you take time to express gratitude for your partner, instead of finding 5 faults, you not only feel more positive towards your partner, you will also experience more gratitude and openness from your partner. You will experience the same positive form of communication from everyone in your circle of family and friends, the more gratitude you show towards them.

Improves physical health

Grateful people tend to experience fewer aches and pains, and they usually feel healthier, and are more likely to take good care of their health. They exercise more often and have healthy eating habits. Improves psychological health Gratitude helps you reduce toxic emotions such as envy, resentment, frustration and regret by increasing happiness and reducing depression.

A positive and grateful attitude also gives you more empathy towards others, thus increasing your self-esteem and helping you appreciate other people's accomplishments.

Being grateful can also help you reduce stress and overcome trauma, as you focus more heavily on the "good" than the "bad".

Better sleep

Studies show writing in a gratitude journal improves your sleep. When you write down things you are thankful and grateful for as the last thing before you go to bed, you have a positive and grateful state of mind instead of stressful input from the tv or your phone.

Write down at least 5 things you are grateful for every night before bedtime. That will make it easier for you to record what you're grateful for each day, vs. just thinking about it.

How Do You Do It

All new habits take time, and writing in your gratitude journal is no different. Patience and consistency are key just like any other new habit. To get you off to a good start, here are a few ideas on how to show gratitude.

Keep a gratitude journal

Write down at least 5 things every night you are grateful for. You can also add pictures and make little extra notes from the day.

Write a thank you note

Ways to cultivate gratitude. Make it a habit to write a thank you card, letter or email to at least one person a month. It makes both the recipient and you happier, and will nurture your relationship

Meditate

Mindful meditation focuses on the present moment with no judgment. Focus on the things you are grateful for such as, the warmth of the sun, a calming nice sound, or something nice someone said to you.

Have an "attitude of gratitude" to create a positive balance in your mind and your life.

Closing

As we come to the end of this "Healthy Made Simple" journey, it's essential to reflect on what you have learned and how it can help shape your life going forward. Use this book as a reference whenever you are in doubt on what and how to make your desired lifestyle changes. Just remember - do NOT change everything at the same time, do it one step at a time.

Throughout these pages, I've had the privilege of sharing not only my personal journey but also some of the favorite things I have learned over years of dedicated study and practice in holistic health. You have also learned how everything in your body, mind and spirit is connected, and how understanding this connection will lead to a happier and more balanced life.

In other words, you need to get back to basics and listen to YOU and YOU only

I want to emphasize that this book isn't intended to replace traditional medicine but rather to complement it, serving as a friendly guide on your path to optimal health.

In a society obsessed with quick fixes, superficial solutions and mixed messages about health and wellness, this book serves as a gentle reminder that true well-being is cultivated through patience, dedication, and good habits as well as finding a balance between modern medicine, ancient wisdom and common sense.

Throughout this book you have learned how keeping things simple can make a big difference. Eating a mindful diet with organic, locally grown, in season foods, as well as letting go of confusion, blame, and guilt, and instead creating a mindset of gratitude and self-awareness all lead to your desired lifestyle.

Ultimately, optimal health isn't about reaching a certain age or fitting into a specific dress size; it's about creating a quality of life that allows you to thrive in every aspect of your being. It's about finding joy in the simple pleasures, nurturing meaningful relationships, and honoring the wisdom of your body's innate intelligence.

As we wrap up, I encourage you to take what you've learned and apply it in your own life. Keep it simple, focus on what matters, be kind to yourself along the way, and continue your journey towards optimal health.

Remember, a healthy lifestyle is a journey, not a destination!

~Ron Williams

Stay Happy and Healthy
Birgitte

Disclaimer

As a dedicated Holistic Practitioner with nearly two decades of experience empowering individuals to transform their lifestyles in simple, effective ways, I am passionate about sharing insights and suggestions for health and wellness. It's important, however, to note that the advice provided in this book is based solely on my personal experiences as well as what I have learned over the years, and should not be construed as a substitute for professional medical advice, diagnosis, or treatment.

It's crucial to understand that I am not a medical doctor, and as such, I cannot diagnose conditions or provide specific medical recommendations. If you have any concerns about your health or well-being, it is always advisable to seek guidance from a qualified physician or other healthcare professionals who can offer tailored advice based on your individual needs and circumstances.

By accessing and utilizing the information provided in this book or on my webpage www.mygoodwitch.com, you acknowledge and agree that you do so at your own risk.

While every effort has been made to ensure the accuracy and reliability of the content, I cannot guarantee its applicability to your unique situation or its effectiveness in achieving your desired outcomes. Therefore, I encourage you to exercise caution and discretion when implementing any suggestions or techniques presented herein.

Ultimately, your health and well-being are paramount, and I urge you to prioritize them by seeking appropriate medical guidance and making informed decisions that align with your individual needs and goals.

Links page

Throughout the book I have mentioned several links and pdf downloads

To make it super easy for you always to have access to the latest version of the book resources, you just need this one link.

www.mygoodwitch.com/bookresources

For cooking inspiration, you can find recipes here:

www.mygoodwitch.com/recipes/

Made in United States
Troutdale, OR
08/08/2024

21848997R00117